*To the health and social care workforce across
the world who today and in the future join
with people at the end of their lives and their
families in supporting them to live and die well.*

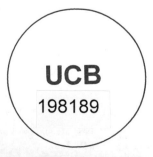

PATHWAYS THROUGH CARE
AT THE END OF LIFE

of related interest

End of Life Care
A Guide for Therapists, Artists and Arts Therapists
Nigel Hartley
Foreword by Professor Dame Barbara Monroe
ISBN 978 1 84905 133 0
eISBN 978 0 85700 336 2

Palliative Care, Ageing and Spirituality
A Guide for Older People, Carers and Families
Elizabeth MacKinlay
ISBN 978 1 84905 290 0
eISBN 978 0 85700 598 4

Spiritual Care at the End of Life
The Chaplain as a 'Hopeful Presence'
Steve Nolan
Foreword by Rowan Williams
ISBN 978 1 84905 199 6
eISBN 978 0 85700 513 7

Speaking of Dying
A Practical Guide to Using Counselling Skills in Palliative Care
Louis Heyse-Moore
Foreword by Dr Colin Murray Parkes
ISBN 978 1 84310 678 4
eISBN 978 1 84642 849 4

Supporting the Child and the Family in Paediatric Palliative Care
Erica Brown
With Brian Warr
Foreword by Dr. Sheila Shribman
ISBN 978 1 84310 181 9
eISBN 978 1 84642 659 9

Communicating with Children When a Parent is at the End of Life
Rachel Fearnley
ISBN 978 1 84905 234 4
eISBN 978 0 85700 475 8

Palliative Care, Social Work and Service Users
Making Life Possible
Peter Beresford, Lesley Adshead and Suzy Croft
Foreword by Dorothy Rowe
ISBN 978 1 84310 465 0
eISBN 978 1 84642 573 8

What Makes a Good Nurse
Why the Virtues are Important for Nurses
Derek Sellman
Foreword by Alan Cribb
ISBN 978 1 84310 932 7
eISBN 978 0 85700 452 9

Pathways through Care at the End of Life

A Guide to Person-Centred Care

Anita Hayes, Claire Henry, Margaret Holloway, Katie Lindsey, Eleanor Sherwen and Tes Smith

Foreword by Professor Sir Mike Richards

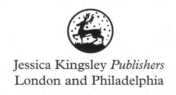

Jessica Kingsley *Publishers*
London and Philadelphia

First published in 2014
by Jessica Kingsley Publishers
73 Collier Street
London N1 9BE, UK
and
400 Market Street, Suite 400
Philadelphia, PA 19106, USA

www.jkp.com

Library of Congress Cataloging in Publication Data
Hayes, Anita Christianne.
  Pathways through care at the end of life / Anita Hayes,
Claire Henry, Margaret Holloway, Katie Lindsey,
Eleanor Sherwen and Tes Smith ; foreword by professor Sir Mike Richards.
     pages cm
  Includes bibliographical references and index.
  ISBN 978-1-84905-364-8 (alk. paper)
  1. Terminal care. 2. Palliative treatment. 3. Terminally ill--Psychology. I. Title.
  R726.8.H388 2014
  616.02'9--dc23
                                    2013023989

British Library Cataloguing in Publication Data
A CIP catalogue record for this book is available from the British Library

ISBN 978 1 84905 364 8
eISBN 978 0 85700 716 2

Printed and bound in Great Britain by Bell and Bain Ltd, Glasgow

Contents

Foreword

When we launched the End of Life Care Strategy[1] in July 2008, the challenge of promoting high quality care for everyone at the end of life was considerable. Over half the population of England and Wales were dying in hospital despite the majority indicating that they would prefer to die in their own home; the number of people surviving into very old age had risen and was predicted to rise even more sharply over the next 20 years yet we knew that people over the age of 75 had significantly less access to hospice and palliative care services; cancer services had shown marked improvements since the Calman-Hine Report in 1995[2] but our understanding of the end of life care pathways for people with other life-limiting illnesses was in its infancy and palliative care services tailored to the needs of non-cancer patients were scarce or non-existent in some parts of the country. Importantly, we knew that many health and social care professionals thought of end of life care as belonging to the last few days or possibly weeks of life and consequently the responsibility of hospices and specialist palliative care services, despite the fact that their job involved the day-to-day support of people who might very well be in the last year of life.

Over the last five years we have seen year-on-year improvement across all these indicators of quality end of life care. This is due in no small part to the work of the National End of Life Care Programme, a small team to which the authors of this book all belonged, charged

---

1   Department of Health (2008a) *End of Life Care Strategy. Promoting High Quality Care for All Adults at the End of Life.* London: Crown.

2   *A Policy Framework for Commissioning Cancer Services: A Report by the Expert Advisory Group on Cancer to the Chief Medical Officers of England and Wales* (1995). Available from: www.dhcarenetworks.org.uk/_library/Resources/ICN/Policy_documents/Calman-Hine.pdf

with supporting the implementation of the End of Life Care Strategy. Through the production of practice guidance, supporting service innovations and disseminating good practice, the team has pursued the National End of Life Care Programme's twin objectives of promoting high quality, person-centred care for all adults at the end of life, across all care settings and health conditions, and supporting people to live and die well in their preferred place.

The degree and scale of change required to ensure that every individual and family can experience a 'good death' cannot rely solely on a top-down strategy and national lead. It requires a culture change amongst the workforce. Across England we have an ever-growing network of health and social care champions[3] who, from the bottom up, work tirelessly to ensure that quality end of life care principles and practices infuse every aspect of care. This book draws on the rich experience and combined expertise of the authors to offer a resource for all those supporting people on their end of life pathway. Its reference point is England, but the themes and issues which it explores are common across the developed world. Indeed, globally we find a remarkable consistency across cultures of what people want when they are dying. They want care which manages distressing symptoms in the most effective way; they want to be treated with compassion, dignity and respect; they want to have the opportunity to set their affairs in order and to be surrounded by those people who are important to them. The implication of meeting those needs, as the core message of this book proclaims, is that end of life care is everybody's business.

Professor Sir Mike Richards
Chief Inspector of Hospitals, Care Quality Commission

---

3   End of Life Care Champions Network: www.hull.ac.uk/fass/eolc.aspx

Acknowledgements

There are many people to thank for their help and support, who have contributed to making this book become a reality. Glenis Freeman has always provided wise counsel and lent her expertise specifically to Chapters 4 and 5. The administrative support team at the National End of Life Care Programme have worked tirelessly with the Programme Managers and Leads in the joint endeavour of promoting good end of life care; their efforts with the many publications and materials that are cited in this book have contributed in no small measure to the establishment of this rich resource. Many thanks are due to Rose-Marie Hetterley for her calm and efficient chasing of references and formatting of the text. Jimmy Turner and Louis Bailey at the University of Hull assisted greatly with literature searches, and Rick O'Brien has driven innovations in social care without which the good practice examples would be much the poorer. The commitment of so many health and social care professionals across the UK to supporting people to live and die well continues to inspire us and we thank in particular those who have provided us with the case study material, which adds so much to the impact of our words. Finally, we acknowledge that the best teachers for all of us are those people who have faced dying and bereavement and used end of life care services in this critical phase of their lives; our deepest thanks go to those who have bravely and honestly shared their stories in the pages that follow.

CHAPTER 1

The Context and Philosophy of End of Life Care

It is only in the last 15 years that the term 'end of life care' has come to be used with increasing frequency. This fact reflects the huge changes that have taken place in healthcare over this period. Palliative care, on the other hand, is a well-established, internationally recognised specialism, an approach pioneered in hospices and transported into other specialist units, which recognises that good care can and should be provided when cure is no longer an option. Palliation, geared towards symptom control and the relief of pain, has made tremendous strides in relieving the suffering of patients diagnosed with a terminal illness. However, it has gradually emerged that the palliative care approach is equally appropriate and beneficial for a large group of people whose condition is not labelled as 'terminal' although it is recognised that they have a life-limiting condition. Moreover, the end of life phase for such people may last months and sometimes years, and the care they require is not limited to relief of physical symptoms, but it is, nonetheless, associated with the end phase of their life.

This shift largely arises from the demographic changes affecting all the countries of the developed world. The UK, in common with northern Europe and large tranches of the US, Canada and Australia, finds itself with a significant and increasing population of older people, most particularly those over the age of 85. Combined with this, advances in medical technology and treatments, including for cancers, are enabling people to live longer, even with serious illness and disease. They may have a range of medical and health, social, emotional and spiritual needs over this period; they may require palliative care as death is imminent; but without a doubt they require care that is better suited to their needs if it takes account of the fact that this person is approaching the end of their life. This book explores these end of life journeys, their unique features and common patterns, and the care and support that health and social care services can offer to ensure that quality of life is as important at the end of life as at any other time. We shall begin, however, by looking at the historical and social context to contemporary end of life care.

The social context of death

The study of death emerged as a new avenue for sociologists in the mid-twentieth century. A growing body of work painted a picture of contemporary death in the western world that became the accepted wisdom for the caring professions. 'Modern death' was depicted as a 'death-denying' culture, with death being shrouded in silence, removed from everyday life and hidden behind the technical barrage and impersonal bureaucracy of the modern hospital, leaving dying and bereaved persons isolated and unsupported (Aries 1974, 1981; Elias 1985; Hinton 1972, 1980). This was often contrasted with 'traditional death' (Walter 1994), the approach to death in simple rural communities in bygone eras, where a matter-of fact acceptance of death in the midst of life and an openness about dying was thought to prevail. Religious rites and social rituals surrounded and sustained individuals in their dying and bereavement and communities found a new place for those whose social status had been changed by the loss of a significant family member (Table 1.1). Whilst this is no doubt an idealised picture of the past, historical accounts lend some credence to it and key elements have become important in the development of good practice in contemporary end of life care.

Table 1.1 Traditional and modern death

Traditional death	Modern death
Death in the midst of life	Death absent from routine/ everyday life
Openness/acceptance of dying	Death-denying society
Dying and bereaved sustained in community	Dying and bereavement lonely experiences
Death accommodated through social and religious ritual	Death technicised and bureaucratised

Social death and marginalised dying

These sociologists described a number of features that compounded the misery and alienation of modern death. First, they pointed out that death is no longer a single momentous event but in fact a series of steps that culminate in the cessation of life, or 'biological death.' Continuing advances in medical technology and life-prolonging treatments have blurred the boundary between life and death even more in the twenty-first century and this presents a number of challenges for the development of good practice models and ethical decision making, which this book will explore. However, not only is dying in a physical sense potentially ambiguous, there are other forms of death that may add to the loneliness and marginalisation experienced by many people as they approach the end of life. Coining the term 'social death', Sudnow (1967) identified a phenomenon that can be as real today as it was when first observed.

Social death occurs when the person is gradually removed from mainstream society. It may be brought about as communication and interaction with the person who is dying become increasingly difficult. It may accompany isolation and the loss of a sense of being useful or valued that is experienced by too many older people. Research more than ten years apart (Froggatt 2001; Hockey 1990) found that care home staff were managing the transition from 'living' to 'dying' for residents in ways that contributed to the dying older person being increasingly cut off. For example, residents were categorised in

Hockey's research as 'fit' or 'frail' and much more recently, Froggatt found the term 'poorly' was used for those residents who had reached the point where it was thought they would not get better. Their care was then managed in this transitional period between life and death by being confined to a controlled physical and social space (Komaromy 2000). The French historian Philippe Aries, who looked at death as a social event from the Middle Ages through to the twentieth century, sums up the cumulative impact of death as 'several deaths' in the modern age:

> Death is a technical phenomenon obtained by a cessation of care… Death has been dissected, cut to bits by a series of little steps, which finally makes it impossible to know which step was the real death… All these little silent steps have replaced and erased the dramatic act of death. (1981, p.88)

It is not insignificant that the hospice movement sought to counter this exclusion of people who are dying by emphasising that dying people *live* until they die (Saunders 1990).

☞   STOP AND THINK!

Could the term 'social death' be applied to the experience of anyone you know of who is supported by health or social care services? What does it take to turn exclusion into inclusion?

Privatised death and the stigma of grief

One of the earliest sociologists to turn their attention to death and dying, Geoffrey Gorer, termed death the new 'pornography' and introduced the idea of the stigma of grief (Gorer 1965). This has been coupled with the idea that modern death has become 'privatised'. The point is not that people necessarily die alone, but that death procedures are taken over by impersonal bureaucracies or professionals and the experiences of dying and bereavement have to be faced without the nurture of a supportive community. Elias (1985) argued that the 'loneliness' of dying occurs when people have to make sense of their experiences alone. Others have pointed to the fact that most deaths take place outside of the person's natural community; some deaths occur without anyone knowing or being involved with the dying person; 'private grief' is regarded as a dignified, civilised process; many funerals and burials are confined to the immediate family, although there may be a memorial service later; and the dead body is taken over by the mortuary or funeral parlour and viewed only by closest relatives if at all (Bury 1997).

Bringing death back into community

Towards the end of the twentieth century, we began to see attempts to reverse these trends. Some writers in fact suggest that this picture of death has either always been partial (Clark 1993; Williams 1990) or that people have developed other notions of dying in community and substituted for religious and traditional 'rituals', symbols and practices which are more meaningful in contemporary society. Walter (1999) suggests that we have in fact replaced ritual with discourse as the 'industry' of grief counsellors has grown up. Seale (1995) uses the accounts of relatives of people who died alone (whether in hospital or at home) to argue that late twentieth-century Britain is very concerned with maintaining the idea that people die belonging to a community that accommodates the deaths of its members in an orderly fashion. Young and Cullen, from their study of terminally ill cancer patients in East London, pursue the idea of 'a collective immortality' (Young and Cullen 1996). They mean by this that there is a sense of continuity between the dead and the living and mechanisms that reinforce a sense of this continuity should be encouraged. This is an open understanding of the fact that life continues in the way it does partly because of the contribution made by those who have gone before, both individuals and passing generations or eras. We see this reflected in the common desire of grieving persons for a deceased relative or friend to be missed and remembered by the wider community. Young and Cullen also emphasised that death contains the potential to 'regenerate morality and human solidarity':

> When all else is stripped away, what remains is a vulnerable human being who can yet be strengthened, even to some extent reconciled by...the feelings of common humanity, and who arouses those same feelings in others. (p.200)

Walter terms this renewed interest in death 'the revival of death' and goes on to suggest that families have 'reclaimed the funeral' and do not need the army of bereavement counsellors that has grown up (Walter 1999). However, there is plenty of evidence that there is much work still to be done in opening up the topic of death and dying, amongst health and social care professionals as well as amongst the wider society and general public. For example, there is evidence that we are better at talking about cancer and palliative treatments or end of life care than about death itself (Holloway 2007). Even hospices, one study found, may be used as places where we shunt away those deaths that are too unpleasant to cope with elsewhere (Lawton 2000) The frequent coverage of death in the popular media is sometimes taken as evidence that as a society we have overcome our reluctance to talk about death. However, these are not the routine stories of death and dying but rather the front-page stories of celebrity deaths, child abductions, murders and mass deaths arising from natural disasters (Pickering, Littlewood and Walter 1997). People being treated for cancer still complain of friends dropping away and wear an uncomfortable wig in a public place rather than face the stigmatising experience of no-one coming to sit next to them because of their appearance. Bereaved people describe acquaintances crossing the road rather than having to speak to them. The need to tackle the continuing fear and taboo of death lies behind such initiatives as the development of 'compassionate communities' (Kellehear 2005), 'end of life care friendly societies' (Walker 2012) and the 'Dying Matters' public campaign in the UK.

Secularisation, religion and spirituality

A core theme in this analysis of modern death is that modern western societies have become progressively secularised. The decline in organised religion is cited as a major factor in the reduction of traditional practices and ritual and, from the point of view of individuals, lack of adherence to established belief systems is seen as contributing to the removal of both a support system and a means of understanding death. There are some contradictory features, however, in this religious/secular debate that suggest that individuals' belief positions are more complex than simply 'religious' or 'secular', and this may become particularly evident in situations of existential challenge, such as facing death and bereavement (Grainger 1998). One study found that dying and bereaved people were conscious of engaging in an existential quest and had a more complex interpretation of the 'why' question than is often supposed; a few were quite specific that where they had sought out a minister of religion it was for his or her experience of reflecting on the fundamental questions that they found themselves facing for perhaps the first time (Lloyd [Holloway] 1997). Another study of people in the last year of life found higher levels of belief amongst them and their bereaved relatives (Seale and Cartwright 1994) and a recent study of funerals reported bereaved individuals expressing a range of specific beliefs about the afterlife, irrespective of whether or not they saw themselves as 'religious' or followers of a particular faith (Draper, Holloway and Adamson 2013). There is no doubt that attendance at religious services in Northern Europe continues to decline, except amongst Muslim populations and some evangelical Christian churches (Voas and Crockett 2005) but a range of attitude surveys have shown that rather more people in Britain claim to believe in some sort of God or greater power than attend church regularly (Bruce 1995; Spencer and Weldon 2012). Davie (2007) has termed this 'believing without belonging'.

Sociological analyses of death have been concerned with secularism and the decline in religion in the west, and anthropologists with the different world religions and their relationship to culturally determined behaviours and 'world view', but the caring professions have adopted contemporary notions of a broader 'spirituality' with rather more interest. There is an already sizeable literature on spirituality and multiple definitions are offered (Nolan and Holloway 2013). However, it would be hard to find a definition that did not contain within it a reference to meaning-making, and in particular the search for meaning. It is perhaps for this reason that the greatest interest in spiritual care is found in palliative care, where the struggle with meaninglessness is often equated with loss of hope (Johnson 2007). It may also be the case that many practitioners are cautious about engaging in conversations with people who hold religious beliefs that are alien to their own, although they will take care to ensure that required religious practices are facilitated, whereas this 'humanistic spirituality' (Nolan and Holloway 2013) can be related to by everyone. The phrase, 'I'm not religious but I am spiritual' has been used as shorthand for a position to which the majority of people today would probably subscribe. Despite this, practitioners repeatedly express confusion, ambivalence and lack of confidence in engaging with spiritual care, although some in palliative care suggest that 'being there', providing a 'compassionate presence', 'helping to find sources of meaning', 'sharing the journey' and 'holding a safe, nurturing space' are perhaps the ways that they provide spiritual care (Holloway *et al.* 2011). Definitions of spirituality also highlight connectedness, relatedness and the meaning found in relationships; this again is a strong theme in palliative and end of life care.

The development of contemporary end of life care

The emergence of what we now term hospice and palliative care arose in response to the pain and distress caused to dying and bereaved persons by the impersonal and often uncaring treatment given in the modern hospital. It should be noted here that excellent medical care was also evident in pioneering centres for cancer treatment, but perhaps the major issue for people who were dying was that the modern hospital was, and largely still is, geared to cure, and death for most medical professionals in the mid-twentieth century represented failure. The work of two pioneers in challenging this view of dying and establishing an alternative approach has been particularly influential. Cicely Saunders, who set up St Christopher's Hospice in the UK, is generally credited with being the founder of the modern hospice movement, but equally important for developing a theoretical framework for understanding the dying process was the American doctor Elizabeth Kübler-Ross. Both these women put their mark on the development of quality care at the end of life, although our understanding of end of life and hence what constitutes end of life care is now considerably different. Nevertheless, the roots of contemporary end of life care can be clearly seen in the revolutionary approach for cancer patients that came to be known as palliative care. Clark (2007) observes:

> In only four decades, the care of patients with advanced malignant disease and the management of their symptoms during the trajectory of illness has moved from the margins

of oncological practice to the very centre of modern cancer care. (p.430)

The hospice movement and the development of palliative care have been extensively written about (e.g., Clark 2007; Kellehear 2006; Saunders 1990) but for our purposes we shall identify four themes/principles that remain critical to contemporary end of life care: valuing the uniqueness of the individual experience; the principle of holistic care; promoting a culture of openness; and understanding the end of life as a journey that ends in death. Taken together, these principles underpin the notion of the 'good death', or 'dying well', which is discussed in Chapter 6.

The dying person as a unique individual

Both Cicely Saunders and Elizabeth Kübler-Ross developed their ideas from listening to, and observing, their patients. For Saunders, the uniqueness of each person and the duty of the carer to nurture and sustain the dying person in a 'community of hope' that did not write them off but rather sought to preserve their dignity right to the end were paramount. Central to her approach was the control of pain, not least because giving adequate and timely pain relief assures the dying person that their individual needs are of central concern to the professional. Being free of the fear of pain also allows the person to concentrate their energies on those things which are important to them, making best use of the time they have left. This principle of care that is focused on the needs of the person in the context of their unique set of circumstances, including and most importantly their family and other relationships, rather than focused solely on treating the disease, remains at the heart of hospice care today and is intrinsic to good practice in every setting or circumstance in which end of life care is provided.

Holistic care

In possibly the earliest articulation of the concept of holistic care, Saunders talked of 'total care for total pain'. In this she implied that the dying person was so much more than a set of symptoms and that their pain should be recognised as 'the suffering that encompasses all of a person's physical, psychological, social, spiritual, and practical struggles' (Ong and Forbes 2005). The concept of holistic care is embedded in good end of life care practice and it has been developed to consider the various dimensions of holistic assessment (see Chapter 3) and the core and different competencies required for all staff to contribute to a holistic approach to meeting need (Chapters 2 and 3). There is, however, a danger that as we break the concept down into its different aspects in order to refine our practice, we lose sight of the fact that holistic care is fundamentally about responding to the needs of the *whole person*, for whom the physical, emotional, social and spiritual aspects of approaching the end of life are experienced simultaneously and as a whole (Holloway 2007).

One way of avoiding this dissection of care is by finding ways of working closely with colleagues in different professions and different care settings. The St Christopher's model of care drew, right from the beginning, on the expertise of a multidisciplinary team that included a chaplain and social worker. There is widespread recognition today that good end of life care potentially involves a huge range of health and social care paid staff as well as volunteers and community groups – 'end of life care is everybody's business' is a frequently cited maxim. More often than not, these people do not work in specialist palliative care but belong to different organisations and sectors and are engaged in end of life care as part and parcel of their wider role. Without the luxury of working alongside colleagues in a tight-knit multidisciplinary team, efforts have to be made to coordinate and integrate the complete package of care. Thus the structures and mechanisms required to provide a holistic, integrated response to individual need are a high priority on today's end of life care agenda (see Chapter 4). The challenge in our complex health and social care systems is to keep the focus person-centred, the system being the means to the end and not the end in itself.

☛ STOP AND THINK!

Is your practice centred on the needs of the person or on running an efficient system? How can those two objectives be brought together?

A culture of openness

An important contribution to the critique of 'modern death' that we have not yet discussed came from the social interactionists. In a study that has become seminal, Glaser and Strauss (1965, 1967) looked at ward life in American hospitals, highlighting the patterns of communication that surrounded people with a terminal diagnosis. They identified four 'awareness contexts' to describe the state of awareness concerning the dying patient's diagnosis and health status (Table 1.2), thereby exposing the secrecy, silence and communication dilemmas experienced by everyone around, and including, the dying person.

Table 1.2 Glaser and Strauss awareness contexts

Closed awareness	*Everyone but the patient knows or deduces that s/he is dying*
Suspected awareness	*The patient has not been told (though relatives have) and tries to confirm her/his suspicions*
Mutual pretence awareness	*Patients, relatives and staff know or decide that the patient is dying but keep up the mutual pretence that the other person is unaware*
Open awareness	*Everyone knows and openly acts or communicates on that basis*

Some 20 years later, the British sociologist David Field studied nurses' and doctors' behaviour towards people on cancer wards (Field 1989). By this time, the communication issues had largely become focused on the practice and ethics of disclosure of the diagnosis. Field found that the diagnosis continued to be concealed from many patients in hospital. Staff justified non-disclosure by arguing that it was for the protection of the patient's ability to cope, but in practice, he observed that they were avoiding disclosure as a coping strategy for themselves. Other research combined to suggest that most people become aware that they are dying at some stage and although substantial numbers of these patients indicate that they want to know, Seale and Cartwright (1994) found that relatives were generally of the opinion that it was 'for the best' when the person had not been given their diagnosis and that professionals preferred to give the news to relatives than to the patient directly. A further strategy employed by professionals was to talk about cancer but not death, focusing on communicating the illness diagnosis rather than its life-limiting implications (Lloyd [Holloway] 1996, 1997).

Out of this position of rather 'fudged awareness' in the late twentieth century, it is now generally accepted in palliative care that there is a moral and ethical imperative to disclose to the person that they are dying (unless they indicate that they do not wish to know) and agreement that open sharing of a terminal diagnosis eases the stress for everyone concerned. Good practice in end of life care seeks to establish a culture of openness and honesty. However, there is continuing unease about communicating 'bad news' and the moral and ethical dilemmas surrounding knowledge of dying, for example, a fear of destroying hope (Twycross 1997). Mortality patterns have shifted and the majority of people now die of diseases of old age such as respiratory or cardiovascular conditions, for which they will not have been given a 'terminal' diagnosis although professionals may have identified that they are in 'end stage'. Many cancers have good survival rates as a result of breakthroughs in treatment and the conversation between doctor and patient may be had in those terms rather than that survival does not necessarily mean cure. Recognising the right moment for each person to discuss end of life care plans thus requires sensitive timing and we know that many professionals avoid such conversations as just too difficult (Chapter 2).

Defining end of life care

So what *is* end of life care? It might be helpful to start by looking at the term 'palliative care', which has been in use much longer, although a 1998 definition from the World Health Organization (WHO) used the term 'end of life care' in much the way that it now defines palliative care. Palliative care is:

> ...an approach that improves the quality of life of patients and their families facing the problem associated with life-threatening illness, through the prevention and relief of suffering by means of early identification and impeccable assessment and treatment of pain and other problems, physical, psychosocial and spiritual. (WHO 1998)

The WHO definition goes on to describe some of the things that palliative care *does*. It

- provides relief from pain and other distressing symptoms

- affirms life and regards dying as a normal process

- intends neither to hasten nor postpone death

- integrates the psychological and spiritual aspects of patient care

- offers a support system to help patients live as actively as possible until death

- offers a support system to help the family cope during the patient's illness and in their own bereavement

- uses a team approach to address the needs of patients and their families, including bereavement counselling, if indicated

- will enhance quality of life, and may also positively influence the course of illness

- is applicable early in the course of illness, in conjunction with other therapies that are intended to prolong life, such as chemotherapy or radiation therapy, and includes those investigations needed to better understand and manage distressing clinical complications.

(WHO 1998)

In summary, palliative care is appropriate when a person has an illness, or is at the point in their illness where the treatment objective is *care*, not *cure*. Its starting point is a medical diagnosis, and palliative *medicine* is indeed central to palliative care; but palliative care also encompasses the psychological, emotional, social and spiritual needs that may accompany a terminal illness.

So how is this different from end of life care? Indeed, some professionals and large sections of the general public (if they are familiar with these terms at all) regard them as one and the same and may use the terms interchangeably.

☞   STOP AND THINK!

How do you understand the difference between palliative care and end of life care?

A much-quoted statement from the US National Institutes of Health State-of-the-Science Conference pinpoints that the difficulties in defining end of life care stem from the difficulties in determining when the period described as 'end of life' begins. The statement goes on:

> There is no exact definition of end of life; however, research supports the following components:
>
> 1. The presence of a chronic disease(s) or symptoms or functional impairments that persist but may also fluctuate; and
>
> 2. The symptoms or impairments resulting from the underlying irreversible disease that require formal either paid professional or informal unpaid or volunteer care and can lead to death.
>
> (National Institute of Health 2004, 2006)

Another definition adds to this picture that '[End of life] is also considered to be the final stage of the journey of life.' In short, 'End of Life is considered to be the period of time marked by disability or disease that is progressively worse until death' (National Institute of Health 2004, 2006).

In the UK, it has become commonplace to speak of the last year of life as the period in which end of life care may be required although it is also recognised that for some people, for example those with dementia or a slowly progressive degenerative disorder, this period may begin some years earlier. In the US, there is greater reluctance to specify a time frame (O'Connor 2008), which some have argued is due to restrictions placed by health insurance companies on care that is not curative (Reb 2003). Others caution against depriving older people of potentially life-saving or life-prolonging technology because they are identified as being in the end phase of life (Kane 2003). Such applications of the concept of end of life are completely contrary to a philosophy of personalised care that aims to enhance choice and promote dignity right to the end.

However, there are good social, cultural and ethical reasons for retaining flexibility around the notion of end of life. Health, illness, ageing, and life transitions – including the relationship of life to death – are variously understood in different cultures and these cultural assumptions underlie how end of life is perceived and responded to (Kellehear 2005). For example, family expectations of the care their relative should be receiving in the final period of life (Brook-Hamilton 2000) may mitigate against palliative care being given alongside life-prolonging treatments. Within our formal care system, older people may be subtly moved from life-affirming categories to a liminal state of dying in which, by dint of being designated as in need of more intensive care, they are gradually removed from mainstream activities, sometimes for several weeks if not months before their eventual death. Thus, there may be advantages to 'blurring of the boundaries' (O'Connor 2008) that allow for a more flexible, personalised approach to end of life care that negotiates between the individual and the system, taking account of personal factors and the family and community context (Holloway 2007). The right time for the 'early conversation' (see Chapter 2) may vary considerably from one person to another.

☞   STOP AND THINK!

In the setting in which you work, who might be approaching end of life? Have they given you any clues that they might be thinking about their death?

If it is difficult to determine when end of life begins, it appears to be even more difficult to agree on a definition of end of life care. In a comprehensive review of uses of the term, O'Connor (2008) explores the way different practice disciplines and clinical specialisms privilege different facets of end of life care. For example, gerontologists identify end of life care as appropriately belonging to holistic care over a relatively longer period that might be termed the 'final phase' of life, while oncologists are inclined to focus on the management of physical symptoms and define end of life care as belonging to the short period when death is imminent. By comparison, social care may take as its starting point that period of increased frailty and debility when the need for health and social care support becomes more intense and the situation less stable (National End of Life Care Programme 2010c). O'Connor concludes that though it is true that end of life care is 'poorly and inconsistently defined' (p.10), a single definition is unlikely to satisfy everyone or adequately encompass the complexities of both the individual's unique pathway and the common care needs associated with certain disease trajectories. While this is true, the authors' experience is that it *is* important to seek a consummate statement of end of life care, in order that practitioners and clinicians across the health and social care network can locate end of life care within their everyday business. Unless end of life care is embedded in routine practice, the goal of quality care for everyone at the end of life will not be achieved. We therefore propose a 'working definition' of end of life care, adapted from a number of sources, which will serve as the foundation for the development of good practice throughout this book.

Box 1.1 Working definition of end of life care

End of life care is the care provided to a person in their final stages of life, which includes but is not limited to the period when death is imminent. It is care that helps those with advanced, progressive, incurable illness or extreme frailty combined with one or more chronic health problems, to live as well as possible until they die. The end of life care phase may last for weeks, months or years. It includes the management of pain and other symptoms and the provision of psychological, social, spiritual and practical support. It is person centred and extends to support of the family and other carers including into bereavement.

End of life care policy and strategy

This gradual development of the field of end of life care is reflected in the history of policy-making and implementing in healthcare systems across the developed world. At the point when the national strategy for End of Life Care was launched in England (Department of Health 2008a), a disturbing picture was looming. We knew certain things:

- Most people die in old age after a period of chronic illness.

- The majority of people state that they wish to die at home (NAO 2008).

- The majority of people were dying in hospital, particularly the over-75s.

- Annual numbers of deaths in the UK were expected to rise sharply.

- Social factors have significant impact on place of death.

(Grande *et al.* 1998; Higginson *et al.* 1999)

This suggested that a broad-based, radical plan addressing all aspects of the care system was required to bring about change. Thus the End of Life Care strategy aimed:

- to bring about a step change in the quality of care for people at the end of life

- to enhance choice at the end of life

- to reduce inequalities at the end of life

- to prepare for the demographic challenge of rising numbers dying in the over-85 age group

- to raise the profile of end of life care amongst both the workforce and the general public.

The National End of Life Care Programme (NEoLCP) was charged with giving a national lead in the implementation of the Strategy, and focused on two core objectives:

- the promotion of high quality, person-centred care for all adults at the end of life, across all care settings and health condition

- supporting people to live and die well in their preferred place.

(www.endoflifecare.nhs.uk)

The National Institute for Health and Care Excellence (NICE) quality standard for end of life care sets out how a high quality end of life care service should be organised so that the best care can be offered. It defines clinical best practice through specific, concise quality statements, measures and audience descriptors to provide the public, health and social care professionals, commissioners and service providers with definitions of high-quality care. It covers all settings and services in which care is provided by health and social care staff to all adults approaching the end of life (abridged from NICE quality standard 2011).

Thus, this is an ambitious initiative flanked by policy, standards and practice drivers, aimed at achieving immediate and long-term change in the quality of care provided to people approaching end of life.

The End of Life Care Pathway

The End of Life Care Pathway used in the UK was first articulated in the Department of Health's End of Life Care Strategy. It provides a framework for care over the end phase of life and outlines six steps in the end of life journey (Figure 1.1).

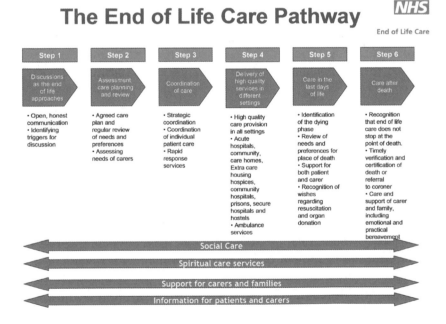

Figure 1.1 The End of Life Care Pathway
Source: adapted from Deaprtment of Health 2008a

The End of Life Care Pathway is a practice guidance tool and as such it is focused on professional roles and tasks and the services required. However, it is important to remember that, as much as there may be common patterns, each person's end of life journey is unique. The End of Life Care Pathway is not a template into which we fit the person, but a helpful tool for providing the best quality care that is right for the individual. People's needs may fluctuate and they may not move through the steps in a prescribed way. The 'oldest old' do not suddenly move from being frail and in need of support to being people who are dying. Clinical pathways conceive of the 'dying phase' as stretching from the point when it is recognised that death is imminent through to the point of death, perhaps two to three days later. Although this dying phase holds true for most people with a serious degenerative or 'terminal' illness, in reality the majority of older people will have been living the end phase of their life for a year or more. They may indeed need palliative care in the final stage of their illness, but for some time before, good quality care will have included consideration of their wishes and future needs as they have approached the end of life.

For some this will have been a gradual process, with their health and social care support needs increasing slowly and almost imperceptibly until a fall or bout of flu leaves them weakened, disorientated and perhaps fearful of what the future holds. Others find their lives dramatically changed overnight following an acute health episode such as a stroke (CVA). Others will have been learning to live with a long-term condition such as dementia, chronic obstructive pulmonary disease (COPD) or congestive heart failure. Good end of life care provides the framework within which decisions can be made together about how these older people want to live this last phase of their life and how they can be supported to die in the way that is 'good' for them.

But end of life care is not just for people who have reached advanced age, although we know that dying in old age with one or more of the common diseases or disorders of old age is the majoirty pattern of dying in the twenty-first century in the developed world (Holloway 2009). For those diagnosed at a younger age with a life-limiting illness or born with a life-limiting condition, early planning for their care in the end phase of life and respect for their wishes surrounding their death, perhaps long before they reach that point, can be an empowering activity – one that validates the person, maintains dignity and enables them to retain a sense of control. Similar things apply to people with a learning disability, who have for too long been excluded from such discussions due to the assumptions of those around them that they lack the capacity and the desire to understand and to engage with issues surrounding death and dying; when bereaved, the grief of the person with a learning disability may not have been recognised, even after a significant loss such as the death of a parent carer.

Routes to success in end of life care

The End of Life Care Pathway provides a framework for understanding and responding to people's changing needs at the end of life. Using the structure of the care pathway, the National End of Life Care Programme's Route to Success (RTS) series of publications offers very practical guidance to help practitioners interpret the pathway. The first Route to Success focused on care homes, and a number of RTS practice guides highlight and address key issues for the delivery of high quality care in other particular *settings*, for example, home care, acute care, healing environments and prisons. Others focus on particular *sections of the community*, for example those with learning disabilities and those who are homeless. A third sequence provides *guidance for specific professions*, for example, nurses, the ambulance service, occupational therapists and social workers, focusing on the particular tasks at each step that belong to their remit. Used together, the End of Life Care Pathway and the Routes to Success facilitate an approach to end of life care that is both tailored to the individual and meets universal quality standards. This philosophy and practice will be woven through the ensuing chapters, each of which is focused around one step on the end of life care pathway.

Conclusion

Death, dying and bereavement in the twenty-first century are experiences that raise complex bio-medical, psycho-social, ethical-legal and cultural issues for health and social care professionals. Yet they are routine experiences for individuals and their families. For all of these people reaching the end of their life there will be families, friends and neighbours who tread this path with them, offering support but often themselves in need of support. Most will not be in specialist palliative care units but in their own homes, supported housing, residential or nursing home care, hostels, prisons – and a significant proportion will end their days in hospital. Thus end of life care, as is often said, is 'for all' and it potentially belongs to the remit of every health and social care worker. The intention of this book is to provide a guide to the knowledge and skills which any practitioner will need when supporting people and their families through the last phase of their life.

Further reading

Department of Health (2008) *End of Life Care Strategy. Promoting High Quality Care for All Adults at the End Of Life*. London: Crown.

Holloway, M. (2007) *Negotiating Death in Contemporary Health and Social Care*. Bristol: Policy Press.

Howarth, G. (2006) *Death and Dying: A Sociological Introduction*. London: Routledge.

CHAPTER 2

Discussions as the End of Life Approaches

Introduction

> It's not easy to talk about end of life issues but it's important to do. Now that we've put our affairs in order and talked about what we want, we can 'put that in a box' as it were, and get on with living one day at a time, cherishing each day together, as I know it's going to end one day. (Carer of person with COPD, National End of Life Care Programme 2010c)

The end of life care pathway begins at the point when discussions about the person's care need to take account of the fact that they are in the final phase of life. This chapter will consider why conversations between the person approaching the end of their life and health and social care workers, as well as with those people who are important to them, are so important. However, determining that someone is at that point in their illness or life course is not always straightforward. Even when a terminal diagnosis has been given, recognising that the individual and their family have taken this on board and are ready and wishing to engage in such conversations requires great sensitivity on the part of the worker as well as skill in opening up the questions associated with reaching the end of life. This chapter will consider some of the reasons why barriers may occur at times that prevent these conversations happening.

A key challenge for staff is knowing how and when to open up a discussion with individuals and their relatives about what they wish for as they near the end of life. Agreement needs to be reached on when discussions should occur, who should initiate them and the skills and competences staff require to take on this role (www. endoflifecare.nhs.uk).

We shall highlight some best practice suggestions and refer to resources provided by the National End of Life Care Programme for England and Wales. These resources identify how early conversations and best practice can be achieved by different professions and in different settings (National End of Life Care Programme 2010a, 2012b, 2013). To aid understanding of the discussion, Tony Bonser's story will be presented in five parts. Tony narrates his experience of communication with professionals, from when his son Neil was diagnosed with cancer and treated up until his death at the age of 35. Tony and his wife Dorothy have worked tirelessly since Neil's death to help professionals understand the importance of timely and honest conversations. Finally, the TALK model is presented (Figure 2.1), which captures the discussion within the chapter and illustrates the steps in conversations for people approaching the end of their lives. This model is intended to aid practitioners to plan and facilitate conversations with people approaching the end of life, and their families, about their hopes and fears for their final years, months, weeks and/or days.

Why have end of life conversations?

Receiving a life-limiting (or terminal) diagnosis can not only be frightening but can also lead to feelings of isolation as people are unsure how to manage their situation or articulate what is going on for them. Likewise, an older person who is aware of their increasing frailty may worry about what dying holds for them, although most indicate that it is not death itself which they fear (Howarth 1998; Cicirelli 2001). Facing this alone, or with a life partner also approaching the end of life, can be a lonely experience. Fallowfield et al. (2002) provides a compelling case as to why these conversations are indeed necessary.

> There is little or no convincing evidence supporting the contention that terminally ill patients who have not been told the truth of their situation die happily in blissful ignorance. A dying person witnesses their deteriorating

body, fatigue and reduction in ability to function. Concealment of the truth is rarely achievable as relatives, friends and HCPs [Health Care Professionals] find it hard not to give out nonverbal clues as to what is happening. The hollow cheerfulness and feigned optimism about quite unrealistic future goals are excruciating to witness, as are the anxious and stressed expressions on faces of people trying to maintain a lie. (p.302)

It can also be suggested that it is the absence of conversations about a person's anticipated move towards the end of their life that is perhaps the most important reason people's wishes go unidentified or unfulfilled. If people do not know how to communicate what they want, or are not encouraged and facilitated to do so, their wishes will remain unknown. Further, if those working with the individual and those important to them do not know how to facilitate these conversations and listen to what the individual wants, the person may be unable to communicate what it is they want and how they would like those wishes to be met.

Box 2.1 You know what you've said, but you don't know what I've heard

'I know how you feel.' I don't think I've ever been so hurt and angry as when that was said to me two weeks after my son died of cancer at the age of 35. The well-meaning friend, whose mother had died the week before aged 94, was trying to empathise and be supportive, but it was just so wrong. Good communication can help enormously to ease the pain of dealing with terminal illness and death. Bad communication can cause anger, resentment, grief and pain which can last for years, and make the process of coping with loss so much more difficult. Professionals can cause as much distress as well-meaning but misguided friends, by lack of sensitivity and failure to understand how their words may be understood.

Source: Tony Bonser, father of Neil

The Dying Matters Coalition in the UK highlights that people and their families can experience a tremendous sense of isolation and can feel shut out of social circles and distanced from their communities (Dying Matters 2013). In addition to feeling isolated by the 'stigma' of their illness, many people in fact are *alone* as they face serious illness and dying. A recent Macmillan campaign, *Not Alone* (2013a), underpinned by research conducted into social isolation and cancer, highlights the even greater need for those health and social care professionals working with such people to provide the support they need (Macmillan Cancer Support 2013b).

Working from the starting point that empowering people to talk about their end of life wishes is fundamental to good end of life care, the UK Dying Matters Coalition, alongside the National End of Life Care Programme and Macmillan Cancer Support (amongst others), believes that a culture shift to promote open, honest communication is necessary for more conversations about end of life to take place. Dying Matters states that it is imperative that people are:

> ...committed to supporting changing knowledge, attitudes and behaviours around death and dying, and aim to encourage a greater willingness to engage on death and bereavement issues. (Dying Matters 2013)

Good communication skills are vital in ensuring that the needs of people nearing end of life, their families and carers are identified, responded to and met. People should be treated with dignity and compassion (Department of Health 2008a). None of this can happen unless conversations are initiated. The Dying Matters key facts illustrate the current situation that underscores the need for this change:

- Eighty-one per cent of people have not written down any preferences around their own death, and only a quarter of men (25%) and just over one in three women (35%) across England have told anyone about the funeral arrangements they would like to have after they die.

- Nearly two-thirds (63%) of us would prefer to die at home, yet of the 500,000 people who die each year in England, 53 per cent die in hospital.

- Nearly two-thirds of people (60%) have not written a will – including a quarter (25%) of over-65s.

(Dying Matters 2013)

☞ STOP AND THINK

How easy do you find it to have conversations about end of life? Professionally? Personally?

Understanding and coming to terms with the diagnosis

Being diagnosed with a life-limiting illness has a significant and life-changing emotional impact. The impact will be unique to each person, as will the meaning they attach to the diagnosis. Therefore the information and subsequent interventions that they will need can only be understood by talking to them. These conversations in turn will enable them to traverse this change in their lives, which some writers have referred to as 'biographical disruption' (Bury 1997). Altschuler (2005) argues that the way an individual moves from being a healthy person to one who is defined as ill does not happen in isolation; rather, it is influenced by factors such as family, professionals and wider societal ideas and issues. Further, no-one but the person experiencing all these factors coming together can identify what 'quality of life' and a 'good death' will mean to them (Sheldon 1997). This underlines the importance of workers listening to the person and easing this transition in the way that is acceptable to and best for each individual.

Kübler-Ross identified five stages that people can move in and out of as they are dying, associated with the gradual and impending losses which attend the dying process: denial, anger, bargaining, depression and acceptance (Kübler-Ross 1969). It is essential for the professional to attune to what it is that the person may be struggling with at a particular moment. For example, if a person appears to be in denial, what specifically are they in denial about – their condition or their prognosis or both? What is it that the person needs in terms of further information or discussion to help them accept their situation? This can be elicited through honest and sensitive exploration of the issues. Many people will naturally feel angry about aspects of their current situation. Again, it is necessary to talk with them to identify what it is they are angry about and establish ways in which that anger may be addressed or managed. Often it can be enough to recognise the unfairness and uncontrollable nature of the situation they find themselves in. Sometimes full acceptance may not be possible at this stage. Can a parent truly accept that they will not see their children grow up, or a 90-year-old fully apprehend that it is time to leave behind a life that has been rich and satisfying? Full acceptance may not be possible, but the health and social care professional's role is to initiate discussions that will enable these individuals to accept that this is the situation they are in and enable them to plan for their care and how they can communicate with those around them in the best ways they can. Anderson (2011) provides examples of common emotional responses following diagnosis:

- *Fear* of physical deterioration/dying, pain/suffering, losing independence, the consequences of illness or death on loved ones.

- *Anger* at what has happened or what may have caused/allowed it to happen, or at unsuccessful treatment.

- *Sadness* at approaching the end of life, restriction of activities due to illness.

- *Guilt/regret* for actions, in some cases for contributing to the development of the illness.

- *Changes in sense of identity*, adjusting to thinking of themselves as unwell/dependent.

- *Loss of self-confidence*, sometimes related to loss of physical functioning/changes in appearance.

- *Confusion* about what has happened, the future and choices available.

It is also possible that people may not as a rule have a good understanding of what their diagnosis means, both now and in terms of subsequent treatments and care options. They may have a previous experience of someone they know dying or have preconceived ideas about a particular illness or what dying means. These experiences will also influence their reaction to their own diagnosis. In addition, many people do not have an understanding of how health and social care services work, nor do they always understand what happens next, what an assessment is (see Chapter 3) or why it needs to be carried out. Therefore, typically they require information and the opportunity to clarify and reflect on this information, bearing in mind that they may be in crisis. Even for an older person, or one who has lived for a long time with a life-limiting condition, the realisation that death may come sooner rather than later can cause significant distress and anxiety.

This is why it is imperative that workers pick up the clues about what they are feeling and listen to what they are saying about their needs now and in the future. For example, it is known that assumptions can be made as to how much and what people actually want to know about their condition. These assumptions do not help the individual or address their need for information and discussions. Shannon *et al.* (2011) cite the Hancock study, which identified through a review of 51 studies that professionals 'consistently underestimated' a person's need for information about their condition and 'simultaneously overestimated' a person's understanding of their prognosis in relation to end of life issues. The researchers propose that professionals should develop a method of communication to continuously check understanding and to keep establishing what information the person needs. It is also important that workers consider how they impart information and the language they use. Factual information or supportive words and phrases may be misunderstood or simply not be 'heard' and received in the way the worker intends.

Box 2.2 Being alert to the effect of words and jargon

Even when the facts are accurate and helpful, the words used can cause emotional reactions, which can have very negative effects. After radio- and chemotherapy, Neil was eventually told by a consultant, 'There's nothing more we can do for you. Go home and get palliative care.' While in one sense this was an accurate statement of the situation, in another, it was unhelpful and ultimately harmful. It was correct that Neil's condition was incurable. However, there was much that could have been done to help him live a reasonably full and pain-free life. He felt, as did my wife and [I], that he had been abandoned. Palliative care meant, for us, 'The end is very near. All you can do is take pain-killers.' 'Palliative' was such an emotive word for Neil that he would not see the palliative care nurse at our local surgery. Indeed he only began to get suitable pain relief when I talked to the GP and explained that Neil would walk out if the word palliative was used. The relief he was given was too little, too late. Professionals must understand the potential emotional effects of their words.

Source: Tony Bonser

Barriers to opening end of life care conversations

There has been much discussion both in the UK and internationally as to why end of life conversations do not happen. There is also a consensus that even if conversations do take place, they may not be in a form that actually meets the individuals' needs (Anslem *et al.* 2005; Baile *et al.* 2000; Bryne *et al.* 2009; Fallowfield *et al.* 2002; Knauft *et al.* 2005; Ngo-Metzger *et al.* 2008; Payne 2012). Fallowfield *et al.* (2002) note that:

> [h]ealth care professionals often censor their information giving to patients in an attempt to protect them from potentially hurtful, sad or bad news. There is a commonly expressed belief that what people do not know does not harm them. (p.299)

☞ STOP AND THINK!

What things inhibit you in opening conversations about end of life care?

A number of common barriers have been identified.

Missed opportunities to initiate conversations

A common problem is that professionals fail to identify either the clinical or social clues that the person is 'ready' and wants to talk about what is happening. There can be a tendency to 'err on the side of caution' or simply not to identify when a person is approaching the end of their life. The result of this will be that an opportunity to open a conversation will be missed. Added to this is a concern raised sometimes by health and social care practitioners across the board that they did not think it was their 'place' to talk about the issues. This again will lead to missed opportunities. People will talk when they want to, to whom they want, if given the space and opportunity. Often people will try to open up discussions themselves in simple terms like 'I wish I had asked the Doctor x, y and z', which then enables the practitioner to follow up with them about 'x, y and z'. Social cues are discussed later in this chapter, but at this point it is important to stress that every opportunity should be allowed to enable a person to express their questions or concerns. From these initial discussions more in-depth support may be given or, if appropriate, referrals to other support agencies can be generated.

Box 2.3 Opportunities for end of life conversations

For me as a daughter and granddaughter I have experienced professionals both taking opportunities and missing them. I am reminded of how when caring for my nanna at home her GP used to breeze in with a cheery 'And how is Peggie today?' until one day he came in and said 'And how are you today?' From that different greeting we were able to have a gentle and truthful conversation as to how I was as the carer. And by him simply reassuring me and informing me 'It won't be long now, you know…', it gave me the strength to keep going and also to ensure people who needed and wanted to be there, were. Also of a missed opportunity, when watching my mum, on the ward in hospital, listening to the St Paul's Choir who had come in to sing to the 'patients' – she loved carols, always had. Suddenly I was hit by the almighty truth she would not be here next Christmas. Not wanting her or my dad to see me upset I turned and went out of the nearby fire exit. As I stood there on the stairs absolutely sobbing, a nurse appeared and simply said, 'You're not allowed on the fire exit' and left. Just at the moment I truly just needed someone to acknowledge my pain, fears and worries as I realised the person I had always turned to previously would soon not be there to do so.

Source: Tes Smith, daughter and social worker

Concern from practitioners that they do not possess the skills

The professional environments in which health and social care practitioners are trained and work have moved away from an emphasis on one-to-one relationship skills to a focus on service delivery outcomes. As a consequence, many practitioners complain that they feel deskilled and ill-equipped to handle what have become known as 'difficult conversations' with people approaching the end of life. In some cases also, the medical complexities leave generalist workers cautious about venturing into a terrain that is not in their area of expertise. However, the phrase itself acts as a barrier as it presumes it will be 'difficult' as opposed to an opportunity to have an open and honest conversation. In addition, these conversations enable important information to be given to the individual to help them make choices about their future care. Managers should engage with their staff and ascertain whether more training would enable them to feel confident to have these conversations with people. There has been much work done in relation to skills and competencies in this area (see Further Reading), though there is as yet little evidence of the effectiveness of communication skills training (Institute of Healthcare Management 2010).

Uncertainty as to how to discuss Advance Care Planning (ACP)

Some workers believe the responsibility for drawing up ACPs (discussed in more detail below) belongs to specialist expertise and as such they will be reluctant to initiate any discussion in case it becomes 'difficult' or 'complicated'. Alternatively, they may believe that someone else involved in the person's care will have, or will already have had, this conversation with them. The fact is that people will express choices and wishes spontaneously at the right time for them, and not necessarily as part of a formal advance care planning process. These are important opportunities to listen, discuss and, where appropriate, record the person's wishes. The earliest discussions are sometimes referred to as 'anticipatory care planning' (Larson and Tobin 2000; Kiehlmann and Williamson 2009) and are equally significant opportunities that should not be missed.

Lack of an appropriate environment

In some settings, such as a busy hospital, it can be a challenge for people to find a suitable place to initiate or conduct private conversations. This can at times constrain what the individual feels happy to talk about and additionally can act as a barrier to workers picking up the clues. The consequences of this are that people may be given information and left to manage its impact alone. Cathy Burgess, former Executive Director and Chief Nurse at Leicestershire, Northamptonshire and Rutland Strategic Health Authority, gave a presentation prior to her death on becoming a 'patient'. A question she posed was, 'Does everyone cry in hospital car parks?' Her experience had been exactly this when, after receiving her diagnosis in an outpatient appointment, she wandered through the hospital alone and back to her car where she wept alone. For the hospital inpatient, it can be very constraining when the person in the next bed is so close or other people's family are visiting, and thus difficult to truly engage in an open and honest conversation about one's future, fears and wishes. Therefore, for those working in places where privacy may be an issue, forethought and planning are critical to facilitating an environment that will be conducive to having meaningful conversations. There is also research that demonstrates that when conversations are had at an early stage in the person's own home, the wishes of the person and their family concerning, for example, preferred place of care and death, have a considerably higher likelihood of being realised (Ratner *et al.* 2001). The home environment was felt to be particularly enabling for minority groups – including same-sex couples and ethnic minorities – for whom fear of stigma and cultural stereotyping or ignorance led to inhibiting of honest conversations in external environments (see also discussion in the Route to Success for lesbian, gay, bisexual and transgender people – National End of Life Care Programme 2012a).

Lack of confidence in managing family conflict

It is not uncommon for families, often well meaning, to have a view that conflicts with that of the dying person as to how the situation is and should be managed. It is imperative to keep the person at the heart of all conversations and plans. In the event of any conflict, workers can enlist the help of colleagues to together support all family members appropriately. Social workers are well versed in managing complex family dynamics and can be enlisted to support or lead family conferences. The skills and knowledge base of social workers equips them particularly well to introduce end of life care conversations and to support people in discussing their wishes and plans, and therefore the role of social work is discussed further below.

Medicalised or clinical bias or use of jargon

It can be the experience for some people that the information that is given to them is very 'medicalised'. For those with little or no medical knowledge, the use of clinical words or phrases may be alienating and may also prevent further questions or conversations from happening. We can all be guilty of falling into familiar jargon or phrases and should notice how we say things and the language we use. This is particularly important at the beginning of the end of life care pathway, as language that creates a barrier may act to prevent the person facing the truth of their condition or inhibit them from asking further questions, both of which have the effect of removing a valuable opportunity to begin the process of working towards what 'dying well' means for them.

Box 2.4 Medicalisation, not personalisation: what does it mean?

When my son Neil was first diagnosed, we were told by a registrar that he had a 50 per cent chance of surviving for five years. I know now that five-year survival is an important measure for clinicians, but for us, faced with the news that our son had cancer, it was simply incomprehensible. Our brains shut down. We just couldn't understand the significance of what we had been told. It was left to a non-medical friend to explain that Neil's chances were in fact either 100 per cent or zero. Statistics which work on large populations, and are of significance to medical specialists, are meaningless to individuals.

Source: Tony Bonser

The evidence shows that communications skills training boosts the confidence and competences of staff responsible for helping identify and meet these needs (Beresford *et al.* 2007; Byrne *et al.* 2009; NCPC 2011; Reith and Payne 2009). A crucial aspect of this training must address how to initiate such conversations about end of life (National End of Life Care Programme 2010a). Is there an optimum time for opening discussions about end of life? It is reasonable to assume that a person will need some level of discussion from the point at which it is identified that they have a condition that will be diagnosed as life limiting. This will mean that from diagnosis onwards there are a variety of occasions when the person and those important to them will need honest and open dialogue. Therefore, those working with individuals and their families need to be able to 'assess' where the individual is and check what information they want at any given time. Fallowfield is clear as to the consequences of avoiding such conversations:

> If HCPs [*Health Care Professionals*] avoid potentially distressing disclosures, patients are not given opportunities

to reveal their own fears and worries and may be left in anxiety-ridden isolation, convinced that they have the most unspeakably horrible fate ahead of them. (Fallowfield *et al.* 2002, p.302)

In this age of a complex mix of health, social care and voluntary services supporting people at the end of life, it is not just health care professionals who must consider this; rather, it is all those who care for and support such people.

Advance Care Plans (ACP)

Advance Care Planning is an essential component of the care planning process. It is about ensuring that an individual's wishes and preferences remain at the centre of support, care planning and service provision. ACP can be a stand-alone process that specifically concentrates on a tool to record wishes and preferences, or it may be part of ongoing discussions with the individual.

> It is important to remember that ACP conversations are voluntary and whilst some of these conversations may be difficult, they are in fact conversations, which assist and can empower the individual. The conversations can help ensure that individuals retain some control, and that it is their own wishes and preferences that remain the focus of care planning. (National End of Life Care Programme 2012c)

The National End of Life Care Programme has developed an online resource called *Advance Care Planning: It all ADSE up* (National End of Life Care Programme 2012c). The acronym ADSE represents the key elements in drawing up an Advance Care Plan: Ask, Document, Share, Evaluate. To summarise:

- *Ask* refers to the need for all those involved in a person's care to ensure the individual is asked and enabled to express their wishes and preferences.

- *Document* refers to the importance of recording the person's wishes and preferences using a standard tool, such as the Preferred Priorities for Care (PPC). Essentially, an individual's wishes can be documented in any form; however, using a tool facilitates comprehensive coverage of specific aspects of care and the wishes of the person. It also enables doctors, other professionals and those in close relationships with the person to know clearly what the person's wishes are.

- *Share* refers to the need to have a system in place so that, with the person's consent, their identified wishes and preferences can be shared with all services supporting them.

- *Evaluate* refers to a mechanism by which the impact and effectiveness of using ACPs can be seen within a locality. Evaluation promotes training and understanding to increase effectiveness in the facilitation of identifying and supporting individuals' choices and preferences.

As with any conversation about end of life, there is no 'optimum' time to have ACP discussions, nor are there only certain professionals that can have these discussions. The discussions should take place when an individual is ready, possibly prompted by any person involved in their care, although it is generally recognised that 'the earlier the better', as this enables the person to have conversations and identify their wishes prior to becoming too unwell to do so. The individual must also have capacity to make informed decisions. In the UK, legislation guides this through the Mental Capacity Act (2005) (MCA), which indicates that a person is presumed to have capacity unless an assessment has found this not to be the case. In the event that a person is assessed not to have capacity to make an informed decision with regards to their wishes and preferences, then professionals will need to follow the 'best interest' principles and process within the MCA (sections 2 and 4). If a person is so unwell they are not capable of contributing to decisions or stating preferences, however, this should not be confused with a loss of capacity. It is important to find a way to elicit any information in the least taxing way for the person; for example, closed questions may be most appropriate at this stage. Family or those close to the individual may also be able to assist with pertinent information. The principles enshrined in UK law are derived from internationally recognised best practice in end of life care decision making where competency is ambiguous or lacking.

It is important in any advance care planning that people are reassured that they can review their wishes and preferences at any time and amend or change them. Some people may not 'be ready' to discuss details and if that is the case, that should be explored carefully with them and a way to revisit some of the issues suggested and followed up. Doctors and other healthcare professionals are obliged to honour a person's stated wishes and preferences where possible. It is also expected that, should the person lose capacity, previously stated wishes and preferences must be taken into account. There may be occasions when family exhaustion and fear of care breakdown may make it more difficult to achieve the stated wishes and preferences. However, where possible those circumstances should not be used to overrule what a person has identified as their preferences. Rather, professionals should work with the situation and the family to implement a contingency plan to endeavor to meet the individual's wishes.

Also, within the UK legislation (MCA 2005, Section 24) there is provision for Advance Decisions to Refuse Treatment (ADRT). Subject to satisfying certain criteria in the way they are drawn up and their application to the specified illness or situation, an ADRT is legally binding. ADRTs are generally used in respect of refusing interventions that are life sustaining and though an ADRT may be verbally stated and recorded in case notes, if it specifically includes refusal of life-sustaining treatment it must be in writing, signed and witnessed and include the statement 'even if life is at risk'. Thus ADRTs are a complex tool in practice and the National Council for Palliative Care (NCPC) and National End of Life Care Programme have jointly produced guidance for the general public and practitioners that deals with:

- how to make an advance decision to refuse treatment, who can make an advance decision, when a decision should be reviewed and how it can be changed or withdrawn, what should be included (in terms of questions or recorded information)

- rules applying to advance decisions to refuse life-sustaining treatment and how they relate to other rules about decision-making

- how to decide on the existence, validity and applicability of advance decisions and what healthcare professionals should do if an advance decision is not valid or applicable

- the implications for healthcare professionals of advance care decisions, including situations where a healthcare professional has a conscientious objection to stopping or providing life-sustaining treatment

- what happens if there is a disagreement about an advance decision.

(NCPC/National End of Life Care Programme 2013)

Box 2.5 The importance of identifying what the person actually wants

Towards the end of Neil's life, when he was in hospital, we visited him one evening. He was lying in his bed, apparently asleep. His consultant came up to us and said, simply, 'I think you should know that in the event of a heart attack, we shall not attempt resuscitation.' We don't know if it had been discussed with Neil. We don't know if Neil heard the conversation, or if the matter had been discussed with him. For us, it was as if the medical profession had washed its hands of him. It doesn't have to be like that. The day before he died, a Macmillan nurse asked him, in our presence, 'Neil, what do you want?' He answered simply, 'I want to go home.' The result was that it was made possible for him to go back to his flat, with all the support he needed. He died a day later, peacefully, where he wanted to be and with the people he wanted with him. This has made grieving so much easier for Dorothy, my wife, and me.

Source: Tony Bonser

Social work and conversations about end of life

Social work is well versed in managing complex family dynamics (Beresford *et al.* 2007; Payne 2007) and, as highlighted in Chapter 3, both generalist and specialist palliative care social workers have a vital role to play in palliative and end of life care, contributing their skills alongside other professionals. In fact, social workers have been in the forefront of developing end of life care practice in many countries around the globe. The UK Association of Palliative Care Social Workers (APCSW) identifies that palliative care social workers are skilled in balancing the needs of those people with life-limiting or terminal illnesses alongside the needs of those who are bereaved (APCSW 2013). The National End of Life Care Programme have also outlined the contribution and role social workers can make (National End of Life Care Programme 2010b, 2012b), summed up by this bereaved husband:

> My children regard [the social worker] as being one of the family. That might not be an entirely professional way to regard her, but none the less that's the kind of impact it's had. (National End of Life Care Programme 2010c, p.13)

Parker (2005) identifies that social workers are all educated in the theories around loss and that social work has contributed to the development of palliative care services. Parker cites Small in identifying three significant themes that have emerged in relation to social work and end of life care. These in summary are that, first, social work has always been aligned to issues around loss; second, social work has a holistic approach with the individual held at the centre of all interventions; and third, that social work in palliative care deals with practical as well as emotional issues. Further, Beresford et al. (2007) provide an overview of many of the areas covered:

> Specialist palliative care social workers offer a wide range of support to patients and families from practical help with housing and accessing other services through advocacy, individual counselling and group support. This will include bereavement work with adults and children both as individuals and in group settings. (p.27)

Thus, their skills in handling complex family dynamics and approaching sensitive issues mean social workers are well placed to initiate end of life conversations. Further, social workers and social care workers, such as home care staff, are often involved in directly providing end of life care. Like their health colleagues, they don't always recognise it as such, or may regard end of life care as the province of healthcare. Ironically, social work as much as any other profession has sometimes to be reminded that 'dying…is not just a health or social care event – it is a human event that needs respect, dignity and support from all' (Smith 2011).

Social workers will also often be involved in the provision of care packages to support people at home or entering a care home. Through this interaction they will by nature be discussing future wishes with the individual and family and the opportunity to initiate a conversation about end of life care is an important one (Holloway 2009). It is, however, important that information and wishes already conveyed to another professional at an earlier stage of care be passed to the social worker making the assessment at the point of transition into residential care. The person needs to feel that rather than repeating themselves because they have not been heard, they have the opportunity to review their plans in light of changed circumstances. This underlines the importance of all the workers involved in a person's care and support ensuring that they liaise and share information, with consent and as appropriate. As the APCSW explain:

> [t]he combination of skills offered by specialist palliative care social workers makes a unique contribution to the psychological and social aspects of the multi-disciplinary professional team caring for patients, their families and carers. (APCSW 2013)

Or as this man, whose wife was receiving palliative care, described, social workers intervene from the starting point of 'conversations with a purpose' (Kadushin and Kadushin 2013):

> [the palliative care social worker] not only understands the patient, and the partner of the patient, she understands the systems as well… It's obvious to us that she knows her job inside out. And just by the way she comes back at you with an answer and what she's saying, you know she knows what she's talking about and that she knows her job and what is available. And if she's not sure, she'll tell you, but she will find out. (Beresford *et al.* 2008, p.1399)

Social clues

Social workers are also well versed in spotting social clues and these will often be displayed alongside the physical symptoms. As described earlier in this chapter, there is a transition for people from being 'healthy' to being the 'ill' person. As the illness progresses and the person begins to accept their situation, they may begin displaying some other social clues as to how they are preparing emotionally for what they are facing. O'Connor refers to some of these as 'ready to go clues' (O'Connor 2008). Identifying these will require listening to verbal clues such as asking about will-writing, or making comments about 'needing to get things in order'. People may also ask obliquely in the form of statements such as, 'I don't suppose I'll walk again' or 'I suppose my travelling days are over.' These are clues to questions they may have and want to pursue, rather than being given an evasive answer such as, 'Oh I'm sure you'll be fine.' Individuals may start offering close family and friends gifts or keepsakes from their home, which can unnerve the intended recipients who don't always know how to respond to the attempted gift-giving. Sometimes health and care workers are likewise offered gifts.

As the person becomes increasingly unwell and moves towards the dying phase they may demonstrate behaviours that again can be social clues. O'Connor terms these 'withdrawal clues' (O'Connor 2008). People may stop reading or being interested in TV programmes or books. Often physical symptoms will increase at this time and they will eat and drink less or show little interest in food. People often stop asking what's happening to those close to them or showing interest in normal day-to-day things. Families can find this particularly hard, as it can appear uncaring. It is important for health and social care workers to notice all these clues, and the family should be supported to understand what this means – usually that the person is disengaging due to the progression of the illness.

End of life conversations with family and significant others

Conversations with the family and those important to the individual will also need careful consideration. These may be had by the staff working with the dying person, with their consent. As Neuberger

(2004) describes, good communication with the individual must always come first, but she further acknowledges: 'Their relationships with family and friends become so important, affect so profoundly how they feel, that to ignore everyone except the patient would be foolish' (p.53).

Brewin (1996) elaborates some of the purposes of these conversations with the people around the individual who is at the end of life: '...[I]n various situations and in various stages of an illness, good communication with those nearest to the patient not only gives them information, it is also a powerful way of giving them courage and confidence' (p.vii).

It may also be that individuals who have been diagnosed will also look for and indeed ask for help in sharing the news with their loved ones. It must be one of the hardest tasks we face to tell people we love bad news. Moreover, those hearing the news will be left with a mixture of emotions with which they may need support. They, too, will have questions, fears and often feelings of disbelief and helplessness. It is not only the person who has been diagnosed who may be crying alone in hospital car parks.

> I could muster enormous strength when visiting my mum
> when she was ill at home or in the hospital. However, when
> I left that visit I knew how the enormity of the situation
> would 'hit me' and I would often stand in a corridor or sit
> in my car and just sob. (Tes Smith, personal communication)

Those important to the individual also need support systems they can access if they are to support the person who is dying. However, offering support to those around the person at the end of life may need careful negotiation to include all parties but also to allow for separate attention to their various needs as indicated and appropriate. A possible plan might be:

• agree whom the individual would like involved – together or individually – and whether it would be helpful to have a professional present to support the individual

• agree what level of information should be shared, and what language and terminology are going to make most sense to those involved

- agree how the next steps in terms of the illness or treatment or symptom management will be explained

- agree to share the care planned now and for the future; this should include the person's preferences for care so that everyone is aware and can ask questions at this stage

- agree on a point of contact or further information for the family members or loved ones

- agree, if appropriate, on a system within the person's support group as to how information and changes may be shared in the future to avoid multiple calls to the ward or carer and

- agree on onward referrals to other systems of support for the family and friends if required.

Good practice in end of life conversations

There has been much discussion as to good practice models and recommendations as to how to approach end of life care discussions with people (Department of Health 2008a; Fallowfield et al. 2002; Knauft et al. 2005; Long 2011; National End of Life Care Programme 2012a; Ngo-Metzger et al. 2008; Shannon et al. 2011). Although each person's situation will differ in terms of the best time, place and approach, all will wish to have information, conversations and support at some point. There is agreement on a number of essential principles on which end of life conversation should be based.

First, all discussions should be based upon the truth. The literature provides extensive discussion of the ethics and practice of 'truth telling'. From a UK perspective, George asserts that honesty should be seen as an ethical requirement (George 2011a and b); Grassi et al. (2000), based on his research with cancer patients in Italy, endorses the importance of truth-telling for professionals. This is far-reaching in its implications:

> Truth-telling also includes being honest about what physicians do not know as well as the inherent uncertainty that pervades all medicine. Telling the truth goes beyond delivering biomedical facts. It also entails humanity. (*The Lancet,* 'Editorial' 2011, p.1197)

George (2011b) acknowledges that truth telling is 'no longer a one-way act of doctors providing information'. Rather, it is a process that enables the individual to express feelings and ask questions in an appropriate and private setting (2011b). Integral to this has to be regard for the individual's autonomy, psychological well-being and social support. Such considerations also encompass issues in relation to a person's cultural background, religious beliefs and in fact anything else that is important to that particular individual and the ongoing management of their illness and their life.

Building on US studies that looked into the need for and implications of truth telling when breaking bad news (Baile *et al.* 2000), the US oncologist Robert Buckman has developed a practice model to facilitate truthful conversations. Buckman's SPIKES model comprises 'Setting up interview, assessing patient's Perception, obtaining patient's Invitation, giving Knowledge and information, addressing the patient's Emotions, Strategy and Summary' (Dennis 2013).

As the SPIKES model outlines, it is important to agree with the person how they would like to receive information and where and how the discussions should take place; for example, who is important to them and how they would like them to be involved. Truth telling, and how it is done, is as important for those close to the individual as it is for the individual:

> Particularly upsetting is watching families, who have not been gently helped to confront reality, locked into stilted discussions about trivia or frozen in silence. (Fallowfield *et al.* 2002, p.302)

The TALK model for end of life care conversations

The TALK model below is suggested as a framework to facilitate best practice in conversations about end of life. It is intended as an *aide mémoire* for practice and to be further built upon by practitioners.

The **TALK** model comprises of the key elements discussed in this chapter:

- **T**ake time
- **A**sk
- **L**isten
- **K**now.

Take time to establish:

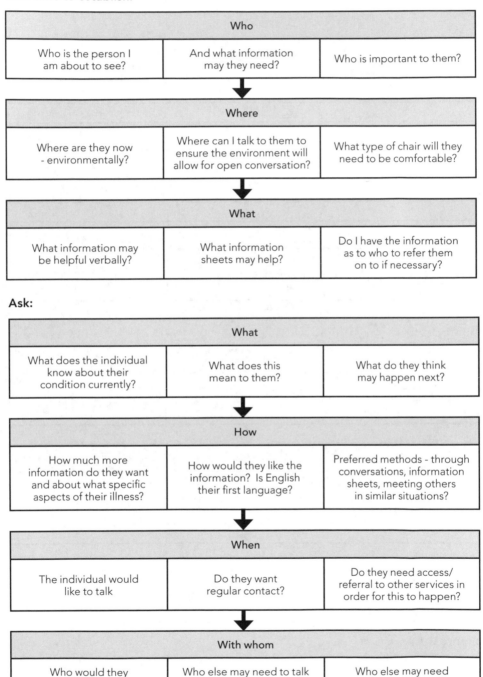

Figure 2.1 The TALK model

Listen:

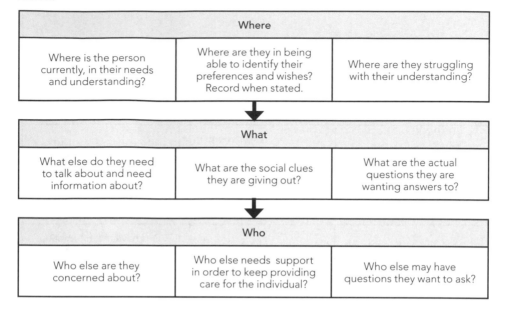

Know:

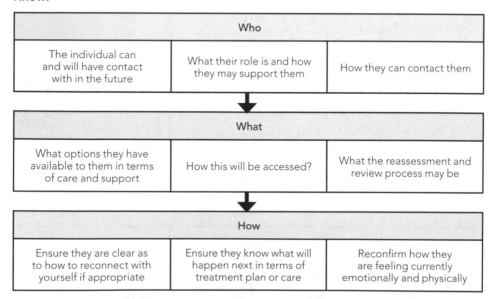

Figure 2.1 *(continued)*
Source: Tes Smith, Social Care Lead, Macmillan Cancer Support

Conclusion

At the heart of conversations with the person at the start of their end of life pathway, and with their family and others important to them, is 'active listening', which hears what they are really saying, picks up the clues about what they want to discuss and registers the unspoken, including social, clues about where they are in their unique personal journey. Key to intervention must therefore be to advocate for the individual and their loved ones as they navigate through the complex health and social care systems.

Linking with all other professionals and care workers who are and will be contributing to the individuals' support is also vital. It is important that all those involved know what the person's wishes are and how they will contribute to the person's care. Information sharing, with the individual's consent, will be necessary to ensure that the wishes the person has articulated are taken into account and achieved where possible. This is particularly important where anticipatory care plans are in place to ensure everyone is clear as to the person's wishes and preferences.

Knowing where the individual is physically and emotionally is just the start of what should be an ongoing 'conversation'. This is unlikely to be a one-off interaction: good end of life care is an ongoing process. Open, honest and truthful conversations as the person begins their end of life journey lay the foundation for all future communications. This includes the person having the information and support to make informed decisions about their treatment options and to have been able to share their preferences for care and place of death. Not everyone will be ready to have this conversation at an early point but it is crucial that there is open communication and shared decision making about the next steps.

As Elizabeth Kübler-Ross pointed out so long ago, it *is* possible to have effective and meaningful conversations with the person at the end of life:

> ...[I]t is evident that the terminally ill patient has very special needs which can be fulfilled if we take the time to sit and listen and find out what they are. The most important communication, perhaps, is the fact that we let him know that we are ready and willing to share his concerns. (Kübler-Ross 1969, p.219)

All conversations, planned or otherwise, must be based in the truth. Well-intentioned skirting round the person's situation does not facilitate good end of life conversations. Nor will it be possible to support those important to them at this crucial stage in their lives.

Box 2.6 Why this is important

I honestly believe that the end result of Neil's cancer was never in doubt from the moment of diagnosis, and that he received the best treatment possible. Communication, though, makes all the difference between a good death and a bad death, good memories and bad ones.

Source: Tony Bonser

People at the end of life need to be seen as individuals and talked to and heard with compassion. They should be enabled to express their preferences and have a right to expect that these will be met where humanly possible. Step 1 of the end of life care pathway is as crucial as any other in supporting people to 'die well', not least because facilitating their meaningful engagement in managing their own end of life ensures that we are continuing to uphold their right to *live* until they die.

Further reading

National Council for Palliative Care/National End Of Life Care Programme (2013) 'Advance decisions to refuse treatment – a guide for health and social care professionals.' Available at www.endoflifecare.nhs.uk/search-resources/ resources-search/publications/importedpublications/advance-decisions-to-refuse-treatment.aspx, accessed 21 May 2013.

Thomas. K. and Lobo. B. (eds) (2011) *Advance Care Planning in End of Life Care.* Oxford: Oxford University Press.

National Council for Palliative Care/National End Of Life Care Programme (2013) 'Advance decisions to refuse treatment – a guide for health and social care professionals.' Available at www.endoflifecare.nhs.uk/search-resources/resources-search/publications/importedpublications/advance-decisions-to-refuse-treatment.aspx, accessed 21 May 2013.

Preferred Priorities for Care (PPC) tools: PPC is a person-held document which was designed to facilitate individual choice in relation to end of life care. Tools are available including documentation, an easy-read version, leaflet, poster and support sheet: http://www.endoflifecare.nhs.uk/care-pathway/step-2-assessment,-care-planning-and-review/preferred-priorities-for-care.aspx, accessed 30 October 2013.

End of Life Care for All – eLearning (e-ELCA) sessions on advance care planning and communications skills. Available at http://www.endoflifecare.nhs.uk/search-resources/multimedia.aspx, accessed 30 October 2013.

Mental Capacity Act 2005, Best Interest process and ADRT (online). Available at www.legislation.gov.uk/ukpga/2005/9/section/2 and www.justice.gov.uk/protecting-the-vulnerable/mental-capacity-act, accessed 30 October 2013.

CHAPTER 3

Assessing Need and Planning Care

Introduction

> The professionals heard and saw what she and we wanted, supported every way they could and mum died at home, with her husband lying next to her, her children by her side and a cat at the end of the bed. (daughter and social worker, quoted in National End of Life Care Programme 2010c)

> The professionals involved in her care should have been involved a lot earlier; then they would have had a better understanding of how the disease was affecting her quality of life, ability to cope independently and the amount of pain she was experiencing... Her treatment was not based around her needs, rather [on] what they thought she needed. She stopped being an individual. (daughter and carer, quoted in National End of Life Care Programme 2010c)

In the previous chapter we discussed those early, sensitive conversations as the person and those close to them realise that they are approaching the end of life. A crucial part of supporting people at this stage is to assess, jointly with the individual and their carers, what their needs are and plan for their future care. Step two of the end of life care pathway should grow seamlessly out of those early conversations and is concerned with putting in place care plans for the immediate and for the future, bearing in mind that those needs will change and that assessment is also an ongoing process. The assessment of need at the end of life is a skilled and potentially complex task that goes way beyond diagnosis of a life-limiting illness.

> An early assessment of an individual's needs and wishes as they approach the end of life is vital to establish their preferences and choices and identify any areas of unmet need. It is important to explore the physical, psychological, social, spiritual, cultural and, where appropriate, environmental needs/wishes of each individual. (National End of Life Care Programme website)

This chapter will focus on how holistic assessments and care planning should be carried out, implemented and engaged with by health and social care professionals working with people approaching the end of their life. It will highlight the End of Life Care Strategy recommendations as to what a person-centred assessment should consist of for those approaching the end of their life. We shall discuss how the domains of a common holistic assessment model may be utilised for someone who has a life-limiting illness and an integrated care plan developed. This chapter will also refer to the importance of integrated working, the barriers to completing a good assessment and the implications of failing to complete a holistic assessment of need for someone at the end of life. The contribution palliative care social work can make in both assessing the individual and the implementation of the care plan will be highlighted.

Why is assessment and care planning important in end of life care?

A cumulative body of work has established the importance of assessment and care planning in delivering quality end of life care. For example, Wright *et al.* (2008) found that end of life care planning improves quality of life for both the individual and their carer. Further, Detering *et al.* (2010) found that the use of specific advance care planning tools not only improves the quality of the care provided but also reduces the stress and depression of relatives in the subsequent bereavement.

A pilot study in the US in which social workers discussed end of life care plans with older people and their families *in the home at an early stage* resulted in 70 per cent dying at home as they had chosen (Ratner *et al.* 2001). In the UK, an evaluation of the use of Advance Care Plans found that they enable individuals to choose their place of death, the people they want to be with them, and support carers through giving them a mandate for decisions made on behalf of a person who may no longer have capacity (IHM 2011).

Commenting that '[t]oo often a person's needs and those of their family and carers are not adequately assessed and addressed', the End of Life Care Strategy for England (Department of Health 2008a) outlines the essential steps making up the assessment and care planning process.

> Individuals must be identified as approaching end of life. The evidence was that people were not being identified early enough to allow for timely assessments and implementation of appropriate care. This frequently leads to unnecessary admissions to hospital, and/or people not being given the opportunity to articulate their wishes for their care at the end of their lives.
>
> 1. Every care plan should be based on an assessment of need. In the absence of individual needs assessment, a meaningful care plan incorporating support tailored to the individual is not possible.
>
> 2. The person's preferences regarding both the type of care they would wish to receive and the setting or location in which they wish to be cared for should be elicited.
>
> 3. The care plan should be recorded with input from the multidisciplinary team. This ensures that both the assessment and care plan are comprehensive and identify ways in which the needs can be addressed.
>
> 4. Services must be coordinated around the care plan for the individual, as without a coordinated joined-up approach there is a risk that the needs will not be met well or that people could fall through a gap in service provision.

5. There should be regular review of the person's needs and preferences and their care plan, as their deteriorating condition may lead to changes in both needs and choices.

6. People should have rapid access to re-assessment and care as their needs change, including access to equipment or additional care support to ensure that people do not revolve back unnecessarily to hospitals or health care provision.

7. A financial assessment should be included within the assessment, particularly in relation to benefits and entitlements.[1]

(Adapted from Department of Health
2008a, End of Life Care Strategy)

In summary, integral to being able to achieve planned person-centred end of life care for an individual is early identification that the person has a life-shortening illness and that they will need to plan for their end of life care. It is only by following a clear assessment process that an accurate identification of an individual's needs can be completed. It is only by identifying these needs that a meaningful and person-centred care plan can be developed outlining how these needs can be met. The assessment and care plan should be seen as an ongoing and proactive process that is both planned and responsive to potential changing needs. Therefore the timing of assessments should take into account changes in the person's condition or circumstances. This is as well as responding to specific requests to reassess or identifying further needs to be met within the care plan from the person approaching the end of life and their families and carers.

Needs of families, carers and those important to the individual

Most, though not all, people at the end of life have family around them and the well-being of the individual is bound up with the well-being

---

1   In some countries this will relate to health insurance arrangements.

of those around them. It is therefore crucial that the needs of family members, particularly those who are acting as carers, be taken into account. In England, carers have a right to an assessment in their own right, and they are referred to in more detail in the End of Life Strategy:

> Carers should always have their views listened to and taken into account. LAs [Local Authorities] have a duty to inform carers of their right to a carer's assessment to determine support needs. The assessment should be reviewed at regular intervals or when changes occur. Carers' assessments should include their physical, emotional, psychological, financial and social needs (including any need for support to maintain employment, participate in education or pursue leisure interests) as well as their ability to continue providing care. (Department of Health 2008a, p.56)

It is important to recognise that it is not just social care services that should inform carers; rather, all those who are involved with the individual and family must inform the carer. Recent research from Macmillan Cancer Support identified that a third of healthcare professionals and 47 per cent of GPs surveyed did not always check what support the person had from family or friends (Macmillan Cancer Support 2013). It is known that many carers do not identify themselves as carers, nor do they ask for assessments and support (Macmillan Cancer Support 2012).

It is therefore imperative that those working with them identify and refer carers for support as appropriate. To ensure that this happens, it is vital that heath and social care professionals work together to identify carers and inform them of their rights, including the right to an assessment and support for themselves to enable them to continue caring. Although attention has been paid to the needs of carers at the time of death and in bereavement (see Chapter 7), greater focus on carers is required at all stages of the end of life pathway if they are to continue to play their vital part in enabling people to die at home if this is the place of their choosing.

Timing of assessments

McIlfatrick's study provides valuable insight as to the fact that there is no identifiable and optimum time to assess an individual and their carers and, additionally, that there is not always a clear time at which an individual's needs are classified as palliative. Indeed, the scope of end of life and palliative care, has broadened to include provision of care at an early stage in the disease's progress (McIlfatrick 2007). This is further supported by the view that end of life is not just the last days or hours of a person's life but rather that planning can start from diagnosis. A prompt that is also now promoted is the use of the surprise question: 'Would you be surprised if this individual were to die in the next 6 to 12 months?' (Weissman and Meiler 2011).

The most important factor is that a comprehensive, integrated and holistic assessment be undertaken at some point. This must be timely for the individual – that is, it is identified that they are currently in need of information, support and services. The responsibility for identification of the need for assessment falls to the professionals or care worker working with the individual at the time. This is where difficulties can occur in that, at times, assessments are overlooked or viewed to be someone else's responsibility in the health and social care 'chain'.

What is holistic assessment?

We should pause at this point to consider what exactly is meant by 'holistic assessment'. The Oxford Dictionary (2013) defines *holistic* as 'characterized by the belief that the parts of something are intimately interconnected and explicable only by reference to the whole'. Perhaps surprisingly to some, it also defines *medicine* as 'characterized by the treatment of the whole person, taking into account mental and social factors, rather than just the symptoms of a disease'.

Therefore the very first three questions for *any worker* approaching a person at the end of life with a view to completing an assessment must be:

- Who is this person in front of me?
- What are their needs in relation to their condition?
- Who is important to them?

☞ STOP AND THINK!

What are my priorities when preparing to complete an assessment?

Holistic assessments for those with end of life care needs, therefore, should encompass all aspects of that person's life. It was this complexity that led the National End of Life Care Programme to develop and to furnish professionals with a comprehensive tool, the Holistic Common Assessment Guide (2010a), which argues that:

> [t]he holistic common assessment process offers an opportunity to explore the individual's wider needs and identify what action should be taken to meet them. There should be a strong focus throughout on supporting choice and decision-making and on helping people identify and achieve the outcomes they want for themselves wherever possible... [T]he individual remains at the heart of this process – assessment should be 'concerns-led' and the process flexible enough to respond to the individual's changing circumstances. (Holistic Common Assessment, National End of Life Care Programme 2010a, pp.6–7)

The holistic common assessment is divided into five domains: background information and assessment preferences; physical well-being; social and occupational well-being; psychological well-being; spiritual well-being and life goals. It is through careful consideration of the person's needs in relation to each of these domains that a holistic assessment can be made and a care plan formulated. However, it is also important to understand that each of these domains impacts on the others and a holistic assessment takes account of this. It is equally important to consider knock-on effects, for example, of physical symptoms on psychological well-being, and to arrive at an integrated assessment of need (see Box 3.3).

Domain 1: Background information and assessment preferences

One of the most basic skills in an assessment is gathering information. Keep in mind that this may be with people who speak another language, cannot speak, cannot hear, cannot see or understand. This domain is to accurately record information relating to the individual in terms of contact details for themselves, family, next of kin, current health care conditions, GP/family doctor and any care services already in place. It is this domain that offers the opportunity to ask the individual what they like to be called (often people are not known by their given name or prefer to be addressed in a particular way). It is also the time in which the family, carer, and support systems can be more constructively identified, and in which the 'who is important to you' conversation can take place. As highlighted previously, people have different lives and lifestyles and it is important to ascertain who it is they want to be involved in their assessment and care plan and who is part of their informal support network. Workers should also avoid language and assumptions that may discourage people from sharing important and relevant information about who they are. Language should be open and inclusive to enable people to feel comfortable to talk openly about who they are, their relationship status and who is important to them. It is important to remember that 'next of kin' may not have legal status (as it does not in the UK) nor does it have to be a family member (National End of Life Care Programme 2012a).

This domain also enables more information to be gained as to preferred communication methods. Identification of any communication differences can be recorded, for example, any hearing, sight or speech issues for the individual and how professionals need to address these to ensure the person is able to contribute fully to any assessment or conversation. This includes the language in which they communicate best and how they prefer to be given information. The reason people cannot access the information may be:

- English is not their first language
- they cannot read
- the terminology used is beyond their understanding
- they cannot concentrate to take in the information
- they are too ill to read and take in written information.

For example, an assessor should not assume any individual is able to read written information easily, perhaps because they have some degree of learning disability; therefore, easily-read information and forms should be made available (National End of Life Care Programme 2011a). Additionally, if the individual or family members are not able to read written English, different language versions of information should be provided. Verbal information sharing should be offered where reading is not an option, due to the person not being able to read or being too unwell to comprehend written information.

Box 3.1 Before carrying out an assessment consider the following:

- What is the current status of the individual's health?
- Is the person dying?
- Does the person still have capacity?
- What is the person's state of awareness?
- What information do I need and from whom and how will I obtain it?
- Why do I need this information?
- What format do I need it in?
- Are there any issues surrounding disability, language or culture that I need to take into account?
- What is the most pressing problem or priority need?
- Are there other people who have vital information and can I gain permission to contact them from the individual?

Source: 'Psychosocial Assessments in Palliative Care checklist,' compiled by Pam Firth and Tes Smith

---

Domain 2: Physical well-being

This domain is crucially important to enable a full understanding of the person's current physical situation and the self-care activities impacting on their daily living routine. This will inform the type of care required to ensure that the person's needs can be met. It is important to understand what is/was 'normal' for that person and what it is that they are finding challenging or that is of concern for them. For example, if the person has not ever taken regular exercise, then asking them how much they do could lead to a false assessment as to their current well-being. The thought behind this is that not everyone takes regular exercise, so if they say they do no exercise this could be normal for them and not as a result of their illness. Essentially what is important is to know what is normal activity for the person prior to illness and whether this has changed recently.

The holistic common assessment offers the following guidance:

> The list of items in this domain is quite extensive and there may be a concern that drawing attention to potential problems might cause worry for some people. Therefore, prior to assessment people should be reassured that the purpose of assessment is to make certain that all potential needs are identified; similarly, it would not be expected that all symptoms listed will be experienced by an individual. (National End of Life Care Programme 2010a, p.15)

Further, the guidance suggests it is important to elicit a clear description of the issue now presenting, its effect on the individual, ways in which they have tried to manage it, or are successfully managing, and what else would help to manage physical symptoms and their impact on overall well-being. If family and friends are providing physical care, this should be identified and recorded as part of the care plan once it has been established that they are willing and able to continue to do so.

Domain 3: Social and occupational well-being

This domain is divided into four sub-domains: managing at home and in the community; work and finance; family and close relationships; social and recreational.

The guide suggests that in relation to each area it is helpful to work through the same sequence of questions in order to:

- ascertain the person's general situation in relation to the sub-domain: *How are things for you in relation to...?*

- ascertain any limits, restrictions or other problems: *What is limiting/restricting you in relation to...?*

- ascertain the support that the individual currently has, and whether this is adequate, consistent and reliable: *What support do you currently have to help with...?*

- ascertain additional support needs.

Approaching the assessment in this way avoids the dangers of making assumptions about people and how they are managing.

Box 3.2 Attitudes and assumptions

Staff vary their approach when they deal with people who they deem to be on the same or different levels of importance. Many times I've noticed the change in attitude to me when people know that I am trained, have a bit of knowledge and am not afraid to speak up for myself... [T]hey feel they are being watched perhaps. This has been marked, around being told my diagnoses. I've had nurses/doctors/psychotherapists/ volunteers/health care assistants expect me almost to 'buck up' because of my training and experience, but some are more understanding because they get that knowledge can be a dangerous thing.

Source: Ann Carroll, occupational therapist and person living with a terminal diagnosis (personal communication)

This domain also records current support from family and friends (informal), or care package (formal) arrangements. It is important to know about support mechanisms, formal or informal, to identify which needs are being met and which still remain to be met. This can also then identify whether these arrangements need to change to meet a new or changing need. It is also necessary to capture any support the person him- or herself currently offers to others such as dependent children, parents or others, that they may be unable to continue to give. This will need consideration in terms of whether referrals to other agencies or social services are required.

Asking a person about their occupation or previous occupation if retired can give valuable insight into many things; for example, are they used to accessing information in written form, are they used to taking or giving direction? Again, assumptions should be avoided; for instance, if someone has a history in the health or care services this does not necessarily mean they either know or understand the situation they are now in.

Domain 4: Psychological well-being

The guide draws on the NICE guidance for supportive and palliative care (NICE 2004) in this domain and outlines the parameters for assessment of psychological needs as 'recognition of psychological needs, leading to effective information provision, compassionate communication and general psychological support' (p.22), making it clear that the need for specialist psychological assessment should be referred elsewhere. The guide starts with the caveat that assessment of this domain should open with a general exploratory question that invites the individual to identify any concerns; it additionally points to the need to be particularly sensitive to cultural differences when asking questions related to mental health. The guide then suggests a sequence of questioning that first elicits a description of the problem, ascertains its history, uncovers its personal impact on the individual and the effect of the problem on others, ascertains the strategies used by the individual to manage the problem and whether these strategies and other treatments are helping and finally asks whether anything further needs to be done about the problem and, if so, what further help the person would like.

Clearly, this line of questioning leads the discussions into a number of areas of the person's life, and for this reason some professions – social work in particular – prefer to talk about *psychosocial* need and support in the context of holistic assessment. Psychosocial assessment and support is essentially based in helping people understand the emotional impact of their illness and/or symptoms.

It aims to work in partnership with the individual and family to identify ways in which they can best manage their problems as well as any further information and support that may be needed. A person's psychosocial care needs are as important as physical symptoms of the illness since, if unaddressed, a person's well-being will be hampered as they progress through their illness. Anderson (2011) provides a guide to some common features of psychosocial care.

Box 3.3 Features of psychosocial care

- Helping people [patients] to understand their options and plan for the future.

- Advocating on behalf of individuals [patients] and those close to them to ensure they have access to the best level of care and services available.

- Enabling people [patients] and those close to them to express their feelings and worries related to the illness, listening and showing empathy, providing comfort through touch as/when it is appropriate, e.g., holding a person's [patient's] hand or putting a hand on his or her shoulder, using complementary therapies such as massage.

- Helping the person [patient] or family member access any financial aid they may be entitled to (including benefits, but also charitable trusts/grants where applicable).

- Providing practical help with daily activities like grocery shopping.

- Arranging personal/social care and organising aids for daily living – setting up a care package, installing hand rails or other adaptations.

- Carer support such as making arrangements for respite.

- Directing the person [patient]/those close to them to relevant resources like local support groups.

- Exploring spiritual issues and ensuring the patient is able to continue his or her religious practices.

- Referring the person [patient] or family member to specialist psychological/social support where appropriate.

Source: Anderson (2011) 'Case report: Psychosocial support for the palliative care patient'

Domain 5: Spiritual well-being and life goals

Spiritual well-being is perhaps the least understood of the domains and exploring spiritual need is the area of holistic assessment in which practitioners in secular professions are most likely to express discomfort or lack confidence (Holloway *et al.* 2011). The Common Holistic Assessment guide makes a number of cautionary statements in relation to this domain and emphasises that it is important to have a 'lead in', 'indicating a shift to questions of a quite different nature from those related to "clinical" needs' (p.24). The importance of being alert to individual and cultural sensitivities is emphasised, as is the question of the different language and terms which people might use, such as faith, belief, personal philosophy, religion, spirituality, personal support, inner strength, personal doctrine. The guide also reminds practitioners that some people may not recognise a 'spiritual dimension' and suggests that exploring 'life goals' enables the practitioner to cover much of the same ground. Whilst this is true, it is also the case that a more common reaction is to regard oneself as 'spiritual' but not necessarily 'religious' (Nolan and Holloway 2013). The HCA guide suggests that it is important first to establish the person's belief position and, as with the other domains, provides a questioning guide to exploring aspects of this (Table 3.1).

In relation to spiritual issues in particular, some health and social care professionals may feel out of their depth. Holloway and Moss (2010), applying the Fellow Traveller Model for spiritual care, suggest that it is important that all practitioners be sensitive to the spiritual needs of the other person and of their significance in relation to the assessment as a whole. However, they should also know when to refer and whom to refer to when they have reached the limit of their own capacity to understand and respond. In actual fact, this principle holds good for each of the domains comprising a holistic assessment.

👉 STOP AND THINK!

How comfortable and confident do you feel in engaging with each of these domains? What do you do about areas in which you feel you lack the knowledge or skills to make an assessment?

Table 3.1 Assessing spiritual needs and life goals

	Guidance for Assessors and Suggested Prompts
Faith/belief	An introductory, exploratory question to determine the person's existing faith/belief, be it 'religious' or non-religious, conventional or unconventional.
Worries and challenges	Identify the person's worries related to spiritual well-being, and the challenges they perceive – e.g., the impact of diagnosis or illness on faith.
Needs relating to spiritual well-being	Identify practical, support or other needs related to religion or spiritual matters – e.g., sacred/symbolic items, a spiritual advisor or support person, spiritual practices and the opportunities to pursue these.
Restrictions relating to culture or belief systems	Practical, support or other restrictions related to person's cultural or ethnic background or belief system – e.g., relating to diet, medicines, treatment options.
Life goals	Person's concerns or desires concerning a 'goal' or achievement – e.g., attending a forthcoming wedding or other family event, taking a 'dream holiday'.

Source: Adapted from National End of Life Care Programme (2010a) Holistic Common Assessment of supportive and palliative care needs for adults requiring palliative and end of life care.

An integrated, multidisciplinary approach

This leads us directly into the importance of working together. Some readers may have felt daunted by the breadth and depth of the holistic assessment process described. You may also have wondered whether it is either feasible or appropriate to undertake such a complex assessment in routine practice with someone at the beginning of their end of life journey; equally, for those who are identified much later, they may seem too poorly to concentrate on all but essential choices about their care.

It is acknowledged that understanding and defining end of life care can be complex. People who require an assessment will be identified at different times, in different ways by different services. The range of professionals and professions who work in the field is extremely broad. Those who may be involved in an individual's care will range from highly skilled and trained professionals to unqualified formal and informal care givers in a range of settings.

What is important in end of life care assessment and planning, however, is that the *principles of holistic practice* should apply across the board. This means that every worker who supports and provides interventions for the person at the end of life keeps the wholeness of the person and their situation uppermost in their mind. The worker's own contribution may be limited to a particular domain, but they ensure that their assessment is integrated with the assessments undertaken by others and that they refer to others' expertise where appropriate.

It is also true to say that definitions continue to be developed and debated as there continue to be different opinions as to the actual boundaries between palliative medicine/care and end of life care (Altilio 2011; Byrne *et al.* 2009; Clark 2007 Monroe 2004). People present with different issues at different times and as such may need access to a variety of professionals and support. The different health and social care services and professionals must work together and good communication systems must be robust to ensure the individual remains supported and, if necessary, is re-assessed as their situation changes.

In order to highlight each profession's role in end of life care many professional bodies have provided guidance for their members who often make up the multi-disciplinary teams that work with those with life-threatening conditions. These are readily found in a variety of sources – for example, in the UK, the General Medical Council

(GMC 2011), the Royal College of Nursing (RCN 2011), the Royal College of Physicians (RCP 2012), the Association of Palliative Care Social Workers (APCSW 2012); the National Association of Social Work in the US also provides comprehensive guidance (NASW 2012).

Not only is the range of professionals broad, the range of settings in which people may be identified as needing end of life assessments is also broad – for example, acute hospitals, community hospitals, the community (mainly in a person's private residence), care homes, sheltered and extra care housing, hospices, ambulance services, prisons and secure hospitals, and hostels for the homeless (Department of Health 2008a, p.79). Once again, in these different settings people will access different members of the health and social work/care workforces at different times. It is crucial that systems be established to share, integrate and coordinate these different assessments and ensuing care plans if the person's range of needs is to be met and care based on holistic principles provided. Failure to achieve this integration can seriously undermine the quality of care received.

> At the opposite end of the spectrum some people are subjected to numerous assessments by different health and social care staff, without apparent reference to records of other assessments. This can lead to frustration and exhaustion, for both the person and their carers, and is indicative of poorly coordinated services and inefficient processes. In addition, it will be important to remember that people with long-term conditions may already have a care plan in place and any plan relating to end of life care will need to be sufficiently flexible to be able to join up with it. (Department of Health 2008a, p.53)

The need for integration is not a new notion for health and social care. It is, however, one that continues to challenge services as to what integration is in reality and how to achieve it. Nevertheless, integration is a theme which runs through discussions of end of life care (Clark 2007; Department of Health 2006a, 2008 a and b, 2009, 2010; National End of Life Care Programme 2010a and b, 2012a and b). Key to true integration is coordination of a holistic, person-centred assessment where all services communicate and work together to provide for the identified needs (see also Chapter 4).

☞ STOP AND THINK!

What other health and social care workers do I engage with regularly? What could I do to enhance the integration of end of life assessments and care plans for the people I provide a service to?

Advance care planning (ACP)

Advance care planning (ACP) is a very helpful tool in achieving this. Its principles and practice are set out clearly in *Advance Care Planning: a guide for health and social care staff* (National End of Life Care Programme 2008). Advance care planning is a process in its own right and can be a stand-alone part of the assessment; however, best practice is for it to be the 'golden thread' through a holistic assessment. ACP is a way of ensuring that an individual can discuss, identify and have documented their preferences for care and preferred place of death as the end of their life approaches. These discussions and the recorded information should be revisited and revised as appropriate as the person becomes more unwell. It is important that the person and their family be aware that the plan is an ideal and although every effort will be made to achieve these preferences, limited resources and restricted access to certain services at times may require a change to the plan (National End of Life Care Programme 2012c).

Linked to Advance Care Plans, though not necessarily included within them, are Advance Decisions to Refuse Treatment (ADRT) – previously sometimes referred to as advance directives. Important revision to these documents has been occasioned in the UK by the Mental Capacity Act (2005) guidance in relation to ADRT. ADRTs can range from verbal requests that are recorded to decisions to refuse all or some specific treatments or intervention which are written by the person and subsequently recorded by the worker. ADRTs are an important part of the advance care planning process and are essentially written directives in relation to specific medical treatment if and when the person becomes unable to make or articulate decisions. Further in-depth information in relation to this is available via *Advance decisions to refuse treatment* NCPC/National End of Life Care Programme 2013) and via the GMC (2011 and 2013).

The UK is, of course, not alone in introducing legislation and guidance in relation to advance care plans applying to end of life and each country's 'directives' will be governed by their particular legislation. However, certain practice principles concerning their implementation are universal:

- Health and social care workers should be knowledgeable, trained and confident to incorporate such measures into their assessments and continuing assessments and reviews.

- They should ensure that individuals and families can access the information they need to identify and discuss what their preferences are.

Barriers to completion of holistic assessments

It is important to be aware of the barriers that can prevent assessments from being adequately completed. For example, workers may feel that they are taking away someone's hope by assessing their current and future needs and thus undertaking an end of life assessment is avoided as a 'difficult conversation' (see Chapter 2). Workers may indeed encounter barriers put up by the person requiring the assessment, some of which may be seated in the person's lack of understanding of their illness and its trajectory, fear of upsetting themselves or others, and ultimately fear of their decline into death. Richardson *et al.* (2005) identify a number of barriers to the effective completion of end of life assessments, many of which continue to be reported anecdotally. Encouragement of reflective practice through supervision will enable some of these barriers to be addressed. In addition, continuous professional development opportunities that address shortfalls in knowledge and skills will support individual workers.

Box 3.4 Barriers to completing end of life assessments

- There is often insufficient time available to complete a full assessment due to pressures of caseloads.

- Lack of sufficient training to complete the tools or understand the processes required to access resources to meet the identified needs.

- The complexity of the multiple assessment tools used means that it takes too much time to adequately understand them.

- Many service providers still insist on their own tools being completed which results in multiple assessments.

- Lack of 'sharing agreements' mean gaps in sharing of information across health and social care services, which in turn results in duplication in assessments and recording as well as lack of sharing of relevant information.

- The belief (and actual reality) that at times the paperwork takes time away from caring for the individual.

- Often the tools are not fit for the purpose, or are not person centred.

- IT requirements affect the assessment process due to the time workers have available to both complete the assessment and care for the individual.

- Workers lack confidence and training and as a result conversations they deem as 'difficult' are not carried out.

Source: Adapted from Richardson *et al.* (2005) *Patients' Needs Assessment Tools in Cancer Care: Principles and Practice*

Social clues

Key to the successful completion of a holistic assessment is the worker picking up on what could be termed 'social clues'. Medical staff and clinicians rely heavily on clinical triggers or physical symptoms as a benchmark for what is happening to the individual. These will help identify when a person is becoming more unwell and also help to at times predict and preempt what treatment will be required next (Ellershaw and Wilkinson 2011; O'Connor 2008). This process constitutes a continuous assessment of the person's healthcare needs. However, running alongside this assessment will also be some social clues which will assist workers to identify what is happening emotionally and psychologically for the person. These social clues will be apparent during the initial assessment phases, and may present as the person not wanting to engage with the assessment process. It is vital that workers look behind the presentation and consider the emotional responses that may be going on for that person which may in turn be causing the barriers (see Chapter 2), since the consequences of not having these discussions are numerous: inadequate care planning; planning not meeting the actual preferences of the individual; carers and families being put under pressure to make decisions for which they may feel ill-informed as to the individuals' wishes. Lack of or inadequate assessment can also contribute to poor contingency planning and crisis management of a situation, when, if end of life conversations had taken place and care plans and asssessments revised as appropriate, a calmer, more seamless access to care could have been achieved.

The role of social work in end of life assessment and care planning

Assessment is a key part of the social work process, as numerous social work writers over the years have attested (Coulshed and Orme 1998; Lloyd and Taylor 1995; Parker and Bradley 2010). Social work has also set great store by its long-standing commitment to the psychosocial approach (Hollis 1972) which some have equated with holistic practice, although other writers suggest that, until recently, neglect of the spiritual dimension seriously undermines that claim (Holloway 2007). Payne (2007) suggests that intrinsic to social work is the role of helping people to improve communications and integration between themselves and the systems or organisations they need to interact with, thus complementing, and helping people to have a positive experience of, health services. It is thus unsurprising that social work is peculiarly well placed to make a significant contribution to holistic assessment and care planning at the end of life (National End of Life Care Programme 2010c).

Early in the history of palliative care, Dame Cicely Saunders trained as a nurse, doctor and latterly a social worker (Cicely Saunders Foundation 2011). This enabled her to utilise the substantial knowledge and skills pertaining to each profession to help her in her quest to solve how to manage a person's total pain. She came to understand the unique role each profession had in supporting the individual. Elizabeth Earnshaw Smith, heralded as a pioneer in palliative care social work, developed the social work role and department at St Christopher's Hospice with Cicely Saunders (APCSW 2012). In a recent interview with one of the authors, she summarised how social work's role was initially recognised:

> I think she [Dame Cicely] gradually realised talking it over, that this [social work] was a different profession that would bring in [its] own professional skills and knowledge. And it would somehow be able to reach out to families thinking about death, to the bereaved families having lost somebody. There was no one in the hospice who did that, looked at the whole thing... [S]he invited me to come and talk about it and it eventually ended up with thinking about having a whole profession that would take it under its wing and work very closely with the doctors and nurses as this was one of the things they did not have at the time. (Elizabeth Earnshaw Smith, personal communication, 2012)

Adams et al. (2009) assert that '[o]ne role of the social worker is to be alongside, to explain and answer questions from service users and carers' (p.89). This is an important aspect for social workers in being able to support those facing the end of their lives, which has been explored more comprehensively by writers focusing on social work with people who are dying and bereaved and the specialism of palliative care social work (Beresford et al. 2007; Holloway 2007; Mason 2002; Monroe 2004; Reith and Payne 2009).

The Association of Palliative Care Social Workers (APCSW), in describing the history of the Association and the role of specialist palliative social work, highlights that, 'social work is an integral part of the multi-disciplinary team within palliative care' (APCSW 2013). Payne (2007) offers a very simple summary:

> So palliative social workers tend to say (accurately) that while doctors and nurses focus only on the individual patient, social workers focus on the family and wider context that affects the patient and their care. (p.72)

Further to this is the guiding principle of holistic practice for specialist social work in the palliative care field:

> Key to specialist palliative care social work is the desire and ability to see people as whole people and not as a set of problems, to understand the connection of their lives and seek to act on, rather than ignore, the constraints and discrimination they experience in society. (Beresford *et al.* 2007, p.27)

The contribution of social work to end of life care assessment and care planning can be summarised in the following checklist in Box 3.5.

Box 3.5 Psychosocial assessment and care planning with people at the end of life

- The individual person should be kept at the heart of the process.
- All information gathered should be shared appropriately with other staff involved and care coordinated.
- A wide range of communication skills should be employed, including the ability to work with translators, use communication tools, etc.
- Appropriate knowledge should be shared with the person who is at the end of life.
- Difficult questions may need to be asked, by both the professional and the service user.

- A person's circumstances and needs should be taken account of in full, including knowledge about their family and/or people who are important to them; 'family' is whoever the person who is at the end of life wishes them to be.

- The trajectory of the illness will have a significant effect on the need to repeat assessments and the cycle of assessment should be adhered to: assess, plan, intervene, review (ASPIRE).

- Maintain a sensitive balance between professional knowledge and an individual's self-determination, recognising that assessment is fluid and an ongoing process that reflects current reality for the person and 'family'.

- Recognise that assessment includes strengths and resources of the individual and their support network as well as problems and challenges.

Source: Psychosocial Assessments in Palliative Care checklist: Compiled by Pam Firth and Tes Smith

Essentially, if a service or professional skill is known about it will be used; should be made in order that people at the end of life have access to the type of care planning and psychosocial support that social work can offer. When people are not linked with and referred to palliative care social workers, they are being deprived of expertise, support and a system that from its inception has been designed to help them navigate their individual end of life journey. Currently, the use of social workers in palliative and end of life care varies across the world, but there is evidence that social work is reclaiming its place and making a valuable contribution to contemporary services for people who are dying or bereaved (Holloway and Taplin 2013). Key to this is social work's contribution to assessment, care planning and holistic, person-centred practice (National End of Life Care Programme 2010a and 2012b).

Person-centred care planning

One challenge for all members of the multidisciplinary team is to keep the person at the centre of all assessments and plans. The individual is capable of making decisions about themselves, their lifestyle and the situation that is right for them. The following case study illustrates how professional views can at times disempower a person from a decision they are more than capable of making.

Box 3.6 Advocating for a person's right to choose

I had worked with Brian, whose discharge home from hospital was seriously delayed by the physiotherapist's insistence that he 'couldn't manage stairs'. Brian was medically fit and desperate to return home to his family and wasn't at risk. The physiotherapist and I agreed that going up stairs was fine but coming down was a risk. As he wouldn't be needing to carry anything downstairs, Brian and I were in full agreement that he was safe and very happy to come down the stairs one by one on his bottom until the recovery process was complete and an optimum lower limb function was achieved. This was based on the Occupational Therapy principle of enabling the person's independence in accordance with their wishes and not with the strict matching of the individual to pure and correct functioning in relation to ADLs.

Brian understood that as his illness progressed his ability would diminish in many ways; he was happy with finding ways to 'manage', but as professionals the physiotherapist and I were not in agreement that the man was safe to return home.

Feedback to the MDT resulted in his discharge soon after the home assessment as the Doctor agreed with me (and probably wanted the bed)! Common sense on this occasion prevailed.

Source: Ann Carroll, OT, personal communication

A significant driver in current UK health and social care services is the policy of personalisation, aimed at 'putting people first'. The plan is that through a significant reform of public services, an assessment through to service procurement/provision system is in place by which people can be given more choice and control throughout. The intention is that people are then more able to live their lives as they wish. Alongside this, people should have confidence that the services they access are of high quality, and that they enable independence, well-being and dignity. Underpinning personalisation is the philosophy of the White Paper *Our health, Our care, Our say* (Department of Health 2006a), which underlines that people want support when they need it, and that they should be able to expect this support to be provided in a timely and easily accessible manner. Key to personalisation is the principle that every person who is assessed as eligible to receive support provided by statutory services or funded by themselves should be empowered to manage their own lives and the services they receive. This can equally be applied to how those living with long-term conditions and life-limiting conditions and those approaching the end of their life are supported in the end phase of their lives.

The Social Care Institute for Excellence (SCIE) has published a guide to personalisation, which describes what is meant by personalisation and the background leading up to it. It further describes the tools of direct payments, individual budgets, and personal budgets which are designed to aid the implementation of personalisation (SCIE 2013). The personalisation of services is essentially being achieved through the development of a system of self-directed support within which people are offered an upfront allocation of resources (cash sums given in lieu of services), often referred to as a direct payment – in other words, a personal or individual budget.

A number of points are critical when considering the use of these tools to support people on the end of life care pathway:

- People with long-term or life-limiting illnesses will have fluctuating needs and individual budgets will need to be flexible to cope with this. Health and social care services must have a robust reassessment/review process. This reassessment must be determined by the needs of the individual and their carers and not by a bureaucratic prescribed timetable. Delays in instigating funding can mean that the support comes too late for people at the end of life.

- If personal budgets are to ensure that people have genuine control over their own social care then informed choice is essential and advocacy services will need to be resourced to support those people who need it.

- Not everyone will choose or have the confidence or resources to manage their own budget, especially at the end of life, so it is essential that the alternatives of directly provided services or that options other than self-managed budgets are available.

- If personal budgets are to succeed for those with long-term conditions or those approaching the end of their life, there needs to be a range of quality and easily accessible services for people to choose from. This includes high-quality information, financial advice and support, emotional and practical/personal care support, end of life care and bereavement services.

(Adapted from SCIE 2013, Report 37,
'Personalistion, productivity and efficiency')

Conclusion

Assessment and care planning for those approaching the end of their life can at times be fraught with barriers and challenges but they are essential steps in the care pathway.

There are many consequences of not completing a holistic assessment. Quite simply, it may prevent the needs of the person at the end of life being identified and the best possible care and support being put in place to address those needs. Further, the person's opportunity to make informed decisions about care planning will be undermined and communication between workers caring for them will be compromised. Most importantly, the individual may not experience a dignified death that reflects their choices and wishes; for those left behind, the experience of their loved one's death could be one of anger and complaint. Simply put, without an integrated, holistic approach to end of life assessment and care planning, we are failing to serve the needs of the person at their most vulnerable. Good assessment practice, on the other hand, is an empowering process that facilitates a dignified end to their life in whatever way is right and appropriate for them.

Further reading

National End of Life Care Programme (2010) 'Holistic common assessment.' Available at www.nhsiq.nhs.uk/resource-search/publications/eolc-hca-guide. aspx, accessed on 25 September 2013.

National End of Life Care Programme (2012) 'Advance care planning: it all ADSE up.' Available at www.nhsiq.nhs.uk/resource-search/publications/eolc-acp-guide.aspx, accessed 25 September 2013.

NCPC/National End of Life Care Programme (2012). 'Advance decisions to refuse treatment – A guide for health and social care professionals.' Available at: www.endoflifecare.nhs.uk/search-resources/resources-search/publications/imported-publications/advance-decisions-to-refuse-treatment.aspx, accessed on 31 March 2013.

Reith, M. and Payne, M. (2009). *Social Work in End of Life and Palliative Care.* Bristol: Policy Press.

Other resources

e-ELCA e-learning

Free to access for health and social care staff and includes over 150 modules covering advance care planning, assessment, communications skills, symptom management, integrated learning, social care, bereavement and spirituality.

www.e-lfh.org.uk/projects/e-elca/index.html

Macmillan Learn Zone

Provides a wide variety of online resources, cancer-specific e-learning programmes and professional development tools, including an out-of-hours toolkit.

www.macmillan.org.uk/learnzone

CHAPTER 4

Coordination of Care

Introduction

> We had two lots of carers. The social services carers came
> in for an hour in the morning and got Mum washed and
> dressed. The other ones, which we paid for, came in for the
> rest of the day and sat with Mum, helped her to eat and
> cooked with her because she'd do things like leave the gas
> on. The carers were superb. They really worked with each
> other too. (Daughter of woman with dementia, quoted in
> National End of Life Care Programme 2010c, p.17)

There comes a point for most people where care may be provided from
more than one source and many people may rely on an increasingly
complex web of care. This chapter focuses on Step Three of the end
of life care pathway and the actions and priorities needed to ensure
that effective coordinated care becomes routine and contributes to
improving the quality of care experience for individuals and their
families. In essence:

> Once a care plan has been agreed [upon], coordinating all
> of the relevant services is essential to ensure the person's
> needs and preferences are met. If a holistic assessment has
> been carried out and shared appropriately, it should be
> possible to coordinate care for the individual, their family
> and carers. This effort may need to involve local primary,
> community and acute care providers, ambulance and out-of-
> hours services, social care, hospices and transport services.
> (www.endoflifecare.nhs.uk)

The NICE quality standard for end of life care in England (NICE 2011) underlines that well-coordinated care should be routine, stating that people approaching the end of life should be able to expect:

> ...consistent care that is coordinated effectively across all relevant settings and services at any time of day or night, and delivered by practitioners, who are aware of the individual's current medical condition, care plan and preferences. (Standard 8)

Once someone has been identified as approaching the end of life and their wishes and preferences have been recorded (Step Two) it is essential that all the different elements of care – and the different services providing that care – are communicated to the right professionals and services are linked together. This is particularly important because end of life care takes place in so many different settings – from hospitals and hospices to care homes, extra care housing, private homes and even prisons or hostels for the homeless. Additionally, it can often transition from one place to another over the course of the individual's last few months.

Care coordination has been defined as, 'the deliberate integration of individual care activities between two or more participants involved in an individual's care to facilitate the appropriate delivery of health and care services' (Bodenheimer 2008). Bodenheimer goes on to suggest that care coordination is required when the continuing relationship between a single practitioner and an individual that extends beyond specific episodes of illness or disease and traditionally ensured continuity is no longer at the heart of the delivery of care. Continuity and fragmentation of care can be viewed as opposite ends of the spectrum; thus, in unusual cases in which continuity is nearly total, coordination is rarely needed. Based on research studies that found that the most common situation is of care where continuity is limited and care fragmented, Bodenheimer concludes that coordination is essential. However, the multiple services that support delivery of end of life care are not always accustomed to talking to one another and sometimes they may hardly be aware of each other's existence. Key challenges arise from the lack of information transfer and communication amongst providers, and between providers, and individuals and their families.

People approaching the end of life are likely to encounter a wide range of professionals and services from all sectors of the care system. In England, the End of Life Care Strategy (Department of Health 2008a) made clear that it is important that these services be coordinated and integrated across health and social care if the individual is to experience a 'good death' (see Chapter 6). The need for joined-up care at the end of life is widely recognised, and some of the best innovations and exemplars are to be found within cancer care. However, in England more than 70 per cent of deaths per annum are not due to cancer and coordinated, integrated care is currently less common for people with non-cancer conditions.

Integrated care models need to be flexible and supported by clear, well-considered protocols and operational policies for delivery. For example, it is increasingly the case that care home residents wish to die within their adopted home – but this requires cooperation and information sharing among care home staff, GPs/family doctors, community nurses, out-of-hours services, ambulance staff, social services and hospitals. In the case of a hospital, an individual wanting to die at home may require the help of a rapid discharge team as well as many support services in the community to achieve their wishes. All these services need to be available and be ready to respond swiftly.

Multidisciplinary and team working

When coordination of care does not happen as it should, the consequences can be devastating for both the individual and their family. Fundamental to getting it right is to ensure a multidisciplinary approach exists, is resourced and operating effectively. The Calman Hine Report (Department of Health 1999) outlined the importance of access to multi-professional palliative care provision for patients with cancer and reviews of multidisciplinary teams in palliative care have evidenced their effectiveness with clear benefits to patients (Higginson and Gysels 2000, 2003). Further, Raftery *et al.* (1996) found that the Coordination service for cancer patients who were terminally ill with a prognosis of less than one year was more cost effective than standard services, due to achieving the same outcomes at lower service use, particularly inpatient days in acute hospital. They reached the conclusion that, on the basis that the observed effects are real, improved coordination of palliative care offers the potential for considerable savings.

There are many examples of excellent multidisciplinary teams (MDTs) working in end of life care, with a large number working in the field of cancer care where palliative care initially developed. The key characteristics of effective multidisciplinary team working in cancer care have already evidenced the importance of having operational policies for how the multidisciplinary team will work. These should include identifying the key worker, the range of people/organisations involved, issues of consent and regularity and format of meetings (NCAT 2010).

Once an individual's care plan has been agreed upon, it is important that all those involved in the MDT are kept updated and that, where possible, they attend regular meetings. Multidisciplinary team working can be real or virtual to enable groups of professionals needing to communicate indirectly rather than face to face where circumstances, such as large geographical distances between services, exist. Equally important is the need to provide support, care and access to advice 24 hours a day, seven days a week. Arrangements must be agreed upon from the outset to ensure that support is available in the middle of the night or at weekends.

Core principles

Given that multidisciplinary teams will operate differently, what are some of the core principles that remain the same?

We would suggest three as a starting point:

1. *There should be a holistic approach* to the assessment of need and delivery of the person's care; therefore the team should consist of all professional disciplines and sectors of service provision.

    Shipman *et al.* (2008) emphasise that it is important to have a balance of team composition and skills. However, the study found difficulties in obtaining this in certain geographical areas, some of which were due to poor recruitment and retention of staff, leading to a lack of skilled professionals.

2. There has to be open, honest communication between everyone involved.

    Higginson and Costantini (2002) compared team assessments of end of life communication in three countries: the UK, Ireland and Italy. Linked to this was an examination of the factors associated with problematic communication between the patient and family, between professionals and patient and family, and between professionals. They found that severe communication problems were reported by team assessments in up to 40 per cent of patients at the end of life, and concluded that a multiprofessional approach is needed in order to make improvements in this area. Curtis *et al.* (2001) highlight also the importance of communication about end of life care during the family conference – which is attended by family members as well as the intensive care unit team. Von Gunten *et al.* (2000) present a seven-step approach to assist GPs in communication when providing end of life care. Step 1 highlights the importance of preparing for the meeting (in terms of confirming the medical facts of the case and ensuring that it takes place at a suitable time and location). Step 2 involves open-ended questions with the patient and family in order to ascertain the extent of knowledge of the patient's situation. Step 3 suggests finding out how each patient would want to receive information, including the right of a patient to decline receiving information. This must be person-centred rather than led by the norms of a person's religious or cultural affiliation and, ideally, should take place from the outset. Step 4 emphasises the importance of delivering the information in a sensitive but straightforward manner. Step 5 highlights the necessity of patience, good listening skills and appropriate emotional responses. Step 6 concerns establishing goals for care and treatment priorities. Finally, Step 7 revolves around establishing a care plan.

3. *There must be clear understanding of accountability* – who is responsible for what, ranging from clinical and practice decisions to direct delivery of care.

    Way *et al.* (2000) define successful collaborative practice as comprising the following key elements:

responsibility/accountability, coordination, communication, co-operation, assertiveness, autonomy and mutual trust and respect. With regards to accountability, the authors state that both independent and shared accountability are important. Shared accountability entails both partners actively participating in decision making and accepting shared responsibility for the outcomes of the care plan.

Evidence suggests a number of features that contribute to effective multidisciplinary working in end of life care:

- ensuring wide representation at the multidisciplinary team meeting

- each service/organisation having the capacity to respond rapidly and appropriately to changes in an individual's circumstances

- streamlined discharge planning from hospital to home with fast tracking of continuing care and support at home

- good communication systems to keep all members of the MDT across all sectors fully informed, including community, health and social care services

- knowing whom to contact in each relevant organisation

- having a structure in place for someone's advance care plan to be updated and communicated

- having procedures in place to support ethical decision making and reaching informed consent.

(National End of Life Care Programme 2011b, 2012d)

This last point is particularly challenging. Kirsch (2009) details the complex nature of decisions at end of life and the conflicts that can occur between a family or significant other's wishes versus the recommendations of the team, as well as the challenges that arise when it comes to respecting, and implementing, patient choice, where possible. Kirsch also draws attention to the multiple needs of the patient, which, they claim, need to be reflected in the complementary skills and disciplines of healthcare practitioners.

☞   STOP AND THINK!

In your experience, what are the enablers and what are the obstacles to effective multidisciplinary working? How are these affecting the quality of care received by people at the end of life in your area?

Box 4.1 When communication fails

James was diagnosed with motor neurone disease in October 2005 and died just two months later. Over the course of that time he had input from many dozens of different professionals and carers, but because of a succession of failures of communication between the different services, that period became a nightmare for James and his family. His daughter Helen said that the biggest failure was around communication: 'The communications and coordination between those caring for my father at home and those in the hospital seemed non-existent. It appeared that notes and assessments from those involved when J was at home, or in the nursing home, were not passed on to the hospital equivalents. Valuable time was wasted re-assessing James's condition.' The result was that all too often it was left to the family to try to coordinate and manage the care her father was receiving. Helen felt let down: 'That really shouldn't have been our role. [Our role] should have been providing emotional and psychological support to our father. There was an appalling lack of communication between all the professionals involved on the health side and between health and social services.'

Below we consider in more detail some of the key components of effective multidisciplinary working in end of life care.

Key tasks

The starting point for this process is identifying an individual approaching the end of life at as early a stage as possible, and then undertaking a holistic needs assessment for potential needs, wishes and preferences as discussed in earlier chapters.

At this stage it is critical not only to develop and record a care plan but – with the individual's consent – to communicate this to all those professionals and agencies that will be involved in the individual's care. Given the rapidly changing, and often unpredictable, nature of the end of life phase, these plans should be revisited and communicated at regular intervals.

This is where multidisciplinary teamwork is especially important. All the professionals involved in the individual's care need to be aware of what is happening.

Roles within the team

Underpinning any multidisciplinary system has to be effective and prompt communication and information sharing across all sectors. At the heart of any system sits the individual and their family. Everyone in the MDT needs to communicate openly and honestly with not only one another but also with the individual and their family, on the principle of 'no decision about me, without me' (Department of Health 2010b).

This means that any sharing of information about the individual has to be done with their consent, ensuring data confidentiality. It is also important to have protocols within the MDT setting out people's distinct roles, who is responsible for passing on what information and who should have access to that information.

Although flexibility and working across boundaries are key elements in successful MDT working, it is also important that everyone know their role within that team and be aware of the limits of that role, and when they should be handing over responsibility to someone else. In addition, all team members need to recognise that this is a significant and often traumatic time for the individual and their family. They should try to offer them emotional as well as physical support in whatever way they can – as well as remembering the need to support their colleagues. At heart this is a matter of showing empathy and kindness. Talking about end of life care for frail older people, Morris (2012) concludes:

> A holistic, humane and kind approach to care underpinned by an effective shared system, communication, education and training and nurses collaborating will ensure more effective care delivery. (p.261)

Key workers

If such a complex web of relationships is to operate smoothly there needs to be a central, coordinating point of contact. In England the End of Life Care Strategy (2008) and the Palliative Care Funding Review (2012) support the idea of an end of life care key worker who can not only coordinate care but also act as the individual's advocate and champion where necessary, whilst offering support and advice. The key worker or coordinator is the individual whom all services can contact when there is an issue surrounding the individual's care; this person should also be taking a proactive role in making contact with agencies such as pharmacy, out-of-hours, specialist palliative care, rapid response services and medical and personal services.

Any worker in the team or network could undertake the key worker role depending on the individual's preferences, local circumstances and resources. For example:

- The coordinator could be the individual's GP (family doctor) since they will automatically be in touch with many if not most of the services contributing to the care package.

- Nurses are often best placed to take on this coordinating role and work in partnership with the individual and their family. They may well be the first people the individual or family approaches to seek advice or raise concerns, so this can seem a natural fit. As the Route to Success guide to nursing and end of life care notes, 'They are often the one who holds the key that fits all the locks and opens all the doors' (National End of Life Care Programme 2011e, p.1).

- In some circumstances social workers may be the best candidates for the role. Social workers seek to give primacy to the individual and their family and ensure their voice is heard and their independence maintained – all things that chime well with person-centred end of life care. They could, for instance, be ideally placed to help individuals and their families coordinate care themselves through personal budgets. They could also take on a more active role should circumstances change.

It should be borne in mind that different elements of an individual's care may need to be coordinated by different people, depending on their complexity. Equally, the identity of the key worker may change over the course of time. For instance, it could be that the most appropriate key worker for someone with learning disabilities would be a member of the learning disability staff but at times when medical issues are paramount, it might be more appropriate for someone from the palliative care team to take on this responsibility.

Challenges

Professionals will often face challenges in understanding and assessing the varied needs of the individual. Assessments can be complex, requiring input from a number of different professionals in a relatively short period of time, especially when an individual's needs change rapidly. Professionals within the MDT need to be involved at exactly the right moment and this relies on clear protocols and communication systems, backed up by contingency plans.

Managing and mediating relationships across different professions with different cultures and expectations can also be demanding. MDTs will also come up against the difficulties of working across boundaries – both within an organisation and from one organisation to another – and of finding common ground between different policies relating to the same issue. All this will require careful groundwork before effective multidisciplinary planning and care can take place. Sturmberg *et al.* (2012) comment:

> The need to think in patient-centred system-wide terms is increasingly recognised… [C]omplex adaptive systems thinking with a primary focus on the patients's need shifts us from questions of 'What is wrong with our health system?' to 'How can the health care system achieve its desired outcomes?' (p.207)

Finally, it is important to bear in mind that these arrangements need to be in place for the whole of the individual's pathway through end of life – which may be years, months, weeks or days. The individual's care needs will continue throughout the end phase of life and the team's resources must be available throughout. This is a moving picture, not a snapshot, and continuity is vital.

Box 4.2 Using a multidisciplinary service to facilitate choice

Macmillan Midhurst specialist palliative care MDT

The Midhurst Macmillan Specialist Palliative Care Service has helped increase choice for those at the end of life and ensure that nearly four in five of its individuals die in their place of choice. The service aims to maximise individual choice by providing as much treatment and support in the home or community as possible. It seeks to avoid unwanted hospital interventions and in individual stays and ensure close coordination between all the agencies involved with people at the end of life. Its watchword is 'Not replicating but enhancing'. Commissioned by the three local Primary Care Trusts and Macmillan Cancer Support, the service consists of specialist professionals as well as a large voluntary team providing active palliative care following early referral from either the hospital or the GP. The service also offers aftercare and bereavement support. An evaluation of the scheme indicated that preventive care over the last year improves individuals' quality of life. Integrated support, including practical and bereavement help, relieves the suffering of both the individual and their family.

Strategies for coordinating care

The 2012 VOICES survey of bereaved people's experience of end of life care in England demonstrated that coordination of care between different parts of the health service and between health and other sectors left much to be desired. Only 35 per cent of respondents felt coordination between care homes and community services 'definitely happened', while one in five said it never happened and nearly a half said it was to some extent only. Coordination between hospital services and GPs and other services beyond was even less evident, and more people felt the services had not worked well together than those who did. The largest proportion (38%) said it had worked well only 'to some extent' (Department of Health 2012c). Similarly, in Canada, Brazil *et al.* (2008) evaluated community cancer services in Ontario and, in particular, gaps in the coordination of services. The study, in part, examined palliative services for those in late stages of cancer. The results revealed the absence of a formal supportive cancer care system and a complex community care system.

These gaps in coordination point to failings not just between people but between organisations. This requires a strategic approach to ensure different parts of the health and social care network are communicating and liaising effectively. That means not only establishing lines of communication between health, social care, housing and benefits agencies, for instance, but also with cancer and end of life care charities and the many other community and voluntary bodies that play such an important part in end of life care. It is also important to have robust handover procedures between primary and secondary care, between health and social care and between statutory and voluntary sectors. In addition, the team should know whom to contact in each relevant organisation and have their contact details readily available. There are a number of examples of coordination strategies to draw on. Harding *et al.* (2010) report on PRISMA – a pan-European coordinating action funded under Framework Programme 7 of the European Commission. Comprising 12 partners in nine countries, PRISMA was designed to promote best practice in palliative and end of life care. Gysels and Higginson (2003) present the findings of 11 separate interventions to improve the coordination of palliative care services. The evaluations were undertaken in the UK (x4), North America (x2), Canada, Norway (x2) and the Netherlands.

☞   STOP AND THINK!

What strategies are in place in your organisation or area that facilitate coordinated end of life care? How could these be improved?

Single access

There are already many examples of successful integration across sectors. The Marie Curie *Delivering Choice Programme* (2013), working with a wide range of stakeholders in the North East of England, has pioneered coordination centres that act as single points of access for organising integrated health and social care services and packages of care.

Box 4.3 Facilitating a multidisciplinary response through a coordination centre

Marie Curie Cancer Care

Marie Curie Cancer Care, in collaboration with local stakeholders, developed the idea of a coordination centre as a single point of access for organising integrated health and social care services and packages of care, thus enabling individuals to be cared for in their preferred place of care. Coordinating health and social care packages can sometimes be lengthy process and a dedicated coordination facility allows clinical time to be reinvested in the delivery of direct individual care. Fully integrated end of life care services can also help commissioners deliver the transformational change required to satisfy the quality, innovation and improvement agendas. Marie Curie has been working to address these challenges with partners in the statutory, voluntary and independent sector through its Marie Curie *Delivering Choice Programme*. In the northeast of England the project involves collaboration between 183 stakeholders (providers and commissioners) across acute and community settings.

Source: www.mariecurie.org.uk/en-GB/Commissioners-and-referrers/Service-design/DCP-Local/DCP-pilots

---

Rapid response

Well-coordinated care depends on careful planning and good working relationships, but it also depends on being able to act rapidly when the occasion arises. Rapid response services in both hospital and the community are essential components of this. Without these, a carer may automatically default to calling general emergency services and the result could be that someone who has stipulated in their advance care plan (see Step 2) that they wish to die at home may potentially end up dying in hospital. They may also spend unnecessary and distressing hours in hospital Accident and Emergency departments.

RAPID INTERVENTION IN THE COMMUNITY

Although some people may move peacefully towards death, others may encounter potential complexity of symptoms and crises which, if not managed with calm and speed, can lead to the individual being hospitalised against their wishes. Coordinated by a central point, rapid response services, available 24 hours a day, seven days a week, are therefore key to ensuring that people can continue to be cared for in their preferred place of care. However, it is important to remember that the coordination of services within the community can be undertaken by a range of individuals or services and that one size does not fit all. In the following examples, one service is coordinated by nurses working with trained support workers, and the other is coordinated by community social care services.

Box 4.4 Rapid intervention to prevent unnecessary changes in care setting

RISE – Rapid intervention service, Oxford

RISE, a rapid intervention service in Oxfordshire, has helped prevent over 250 emergency admissions in its first year. Over the course of a year the team prevented 258 emergency admissions while admitting just 26 patients. One of the keys to success has been close coordination with other services. The service is staffed by a Registered General Nurse, who does the initial assessment of needs and care plan, together with a team of trained support workers. Another trained nurse acts as coordinator and staffs a dedicated telephone helpline. The team aims either to refer each individual on to the appropriate service or to support the individual and family until the time of death. At times of crisis it seeks to make contact within 20 minutes. A big emphasis is placed on close coordination with other services such as the GP Fast Track Team and key worker.

Cumbria – A Rapid Response Social Care team

In Cumbria a group of specially trained home care staff, managed by adult services social workers, are responsible for supporting people at the end of life. They have a network of close and supportive relationships with preferred care agencies – including a rapid response team – to ensure they are able to provide appropriate and immediate care when needed. Key to this process, which is proving very successful, is careful sharing of information. Staff are encouraged to look out for and report back to social workers any unmet needs or emerging concerns.

RAPID DISCHARGE FROM HOSPITAL

Many hospitals have now set up arrangements that allow people to be discharged to their home within 24 or 48 hours and a number are working towards discharge within a matter of hours. These pathways are usually combined partnerships among district/community nurses, GPs, ambulance services, hospices and social care as well as equipment services and hospital teams. Each of these key services should have input since each will need to work out how their working practice fits in with the pathway. For example, some district/community nursing services will not look after people at the end of life without a hospital bed being in the home, so plans would need to be in place for this. The following need to be considered:

- Handover of medication is essential, so good documentation is needed using local prescription formats to ensure that medications started in hospital can be given by community nursing staff without having to wait for GPs to prescribe.

- It is useful to have an end of life care discharge checklist in place highlighting relevant information for community teams such as 'Do not Attempt Cardio-Pulmonary Resuscitation' directives (DNACPR), preferred place of care and advance care planning.

- It is important to be able to fast track funding streams (for example, in England to be able to fast-track NHS continuing health care funding) and to ensure appropriate support is available in the individual's home.

- Sensitive discussions need to take place with individuals and their families about the risks of transporting someone who is at an advanced stage of their illness.

Box 4.5 Enabling the choice to die at home

Robert was at the end of life but desperate to go home and see his garden before he died. Staff worked feverishly to get him home but he was so frail they were worried he might not survive the journey. In the event they got him back and three hours later his wife phoned to say he had died. The discharge facilitator on the case said, 'To them it meant everything that he was at home when it happened and to me I'll always feel that was worthwhile.'

Mechanisms for coordinating care

The aim of fully coordinated end of life care is straightforward: ensuring that the right care is provided to the individual at the right time and in the right place. However, making this happen is a complex and multi-faceted task and a number of mechanisms have been developed to facilitate the process.

Anticipatory medication

It is important to have plans in place for that moment when an immediate treatment response is required. This would include the ability to bring in equipment such as special mattresses at short notice but staff should also have rapid access to medication either through arrangements with local pharmacies or by having anticipatory medication in the home. Faull *et al.* (2012) acknowledge that anticipatory prescribing is key to ensuring high-quality end of life care. They explore the challenges encountered by community health professionals in Leicestershire and Rutland with regards to anticipatory prescribing when caring for terminally ill patients who wish to die at home. The study found that professionals' relationships with other professionals presented challenges, as did links between community and hospital care providers – especially between 'usual' and 'out-of-hours' care providers. The authors highlight the importance of building and maintaining good communication and trust between professional teams and working practices.

One model used in England that is proving very successful is the 'Just in Case' boxes, which contain a range of medication prescribed in advance by the GP or specialist nurse and are lodged in a safe place in the home. The 'Gold Standards Framework Examples of

Good Practice Resource Guide' (2006) sets out information to assist in developing 'Just in Case' boxes in the local area and guidance on content of the boxes. Other pre-emptive prescribing mechanisms include 'Breathing Space boxes' – which are designed for patients with end-stage motor neurone disease (MND) at risk of severe breathlessness, panic or choking; palliative care emergency kits, which generally include a wider range of prescription drugs than a Just in Case box; and extended pharmacy schemes, which offer extended opening hours and carry extended palliative care stock.

Box 4.6 Supporting early hospital discharge with anticipatory medication

North Staffs hospital discharge scheme

A rapid discharge pathway at the University Hospital of North Staffordshire is enabling end of life care individuals to be discharged within days or even hours. Around 45 individuals each quarter are now being fast-tracked in this way. The process is triggered when an individual is identified as possibly being in the last weeks or months of life and wishing to go home or to an alternative place of care.

Strong working relationships have developed between teams. This extends across the secondary and primary care divide, with new services being developed to support individuals dying in their preferred place of care. The ward team responsible for the individual's care will discuss the plan of care and likely prognosis with the individual and family according to individual need. The team also refers the individual to the hospital complex assessment team and the palliative occupational therapist within a maximum of two hours. The plan, funding and care package is coordinated by the complex assessment nurse who liaises with the individual, family and multidisciplinary team both in the hospital and community. The discharge is then arranged at the earliest possible opportunity. A number of tools to support staff have been developed including a pro forma for anticipatory prescribing of end of life care take-home medications, a palliative and end of life care discharge checklist and an end of life care 'flagging' on the hospital IT system, which generates a letter to the GP to highlight the person's palliative care needs.

Electronic coordinating systems

Given the diversity of organisations and agencies across settings involved in coordinating good end of life care, the development of electronic systems is an important tool to enable easier communication, transfer and sharing of information. Electronic information-sharing of a person's wishes, preferences and current health status and social situation can help to keep all the involved organisations and agencies in the loop and so ensure the person receives the right support at the right time.

Several electronic systems to coordinate end of life care are already operating successfully in the United States. Claiming that Health Information Technology (HIT) is underused by hospice and palliative care organisations in the US, Abernethy et al. (2011) developed an HIT-based data infrastructure. The network was pilot-tested at a community-based site then refined and analysed, with a view to being rolled out across additional sites. The project encouraged buy-in via the recruitment of site-based champions, local community engagement and a consortium approach of joined-up thinking. As a result of this project, electronic data collection proved to be feasible and desired within the area of hospice and palliative care. Elsewhere, Buntin et al. (2011) found that 92 per cent of articles on Health Information Technology (HIT) in the US reported favourable outcomes in relation to quality, efficiency and service provider satisfaction. However, the authors found that there are still small pockets of dissatisfaction with electronic records. The costs and challenges of implementing electronic health records are explored in greater depth by Fleming (2011).

In England a number of sites are now using Electronic Palliative Care Coordination Systems (EPaCCS) and a similar system, entitled the electronic Palliative Care Summary (ePCS), operates in Scotland. EPaCCS developed in England between 2009 and 2012. The aim is to provide a single point where all relevant information about an individual can be recorded and then shared with all those who need to know. This has to be undertaken with the individual's consent. Prior to the introduction of EPaCCS, pilots testing different approaches to electronic registers were undertaken between 2009 and 2011 to ensure they supported early identification of people approaching the end of life and contributed to the appropriate planning of their care.

The early evidence from sites using EPaCCS suggested the system helped more people to achieve their wishes and preferences enabling them to die in their usual place of residence. A survey undertaken in 2012 across nine sites using EPaCCS (National End of Life Care Programme 2012e) showed that deaths in hospital were around a third of the national average while deaths at home and in hospices were more than twice the national average. For one site, 80 per cent of those on a register who expressed a preference for place of death, and had their wishes concerning actual place of death recorded, achieved their wish. By 2012, a total of 25,177 people were on EPaCCS, accounting for one in seven of all deaths in the areas covered. Of those on the system 3950 are reported as having recorded their preferred place of death, with 1502 (38%) having achieved that to date. In Scotland, Smith and Sherwin (2012) investigated whether the EPaCCS improved the quality of information shared compared with the previous Faxed Palliative Care Handover Forms (PCHF) that it replaced. They found that EPaCCS has improved the quality of data inputted and consequently shared.

Box 4.7 Facilitating preferred place of care through electronic communication

Norman, a man in his 80s with fibrosing alveolitis, decided he did not want to be admitted to hospital again unless it was unavoidable and would refuse any further 'heroic' treatment. He also said he would prefer to die in a hospice rather than at home because he felt it would be too much for his wife. A week later Norman had an unexpected crisis and because his details and wishes had been recorded on EPaCCS, out-of-hours medical and healthcare staff knew what he wanted and a bed was found for him at the local hospice. One month later he died there with his wife at his bedside. Norman's clinical nurse specialist in palliative care was glad she had been able to record Norman's last wishes before it was too late and that the system was in place to retrieve those wishes in the crisis: 'It makes such a difference to know what someone wants at the end of their life rather than just making assumptions,' she said. She had little doubt that if Norman and his wife hadn't had that conversation at the clinic, he would have ended up in hospital against his wishes. His wife also believes that establishing Norman's wishes in advance and making sure they were respected made a big difference not only to his immediate care but to how the family were able to grieve afterwards: 'Getting that right does help the immediate grieving process because you aren't full of regrets that can get in the way of other things.'

Evaluations of EPaCCS (Ipsos Mori 2011; National End of Life Care Programme 2012f) also point to improved patient experiences across a range of measures. Better communication among the different services involved in end of life care resulted in reductions in unnecessary interventions and fewer inappropriate emergency hospital admissions. Patients also benefited from:

- improved communication between professionals with more clarity of staff involved and how to contact them

- improved access to key information that is not otherwise available e.g., for ambulance staff and out-of-hours providers

- improved communication of Advance Decision to Refuse Treatment, Do Not Attempt Cardio-Pulmonary Resuscitation decisions and advance statements of wishes and preferences

- improved communication of the issue and location of anticipatory medication

- clarity of people involved in the care who should be involved in decision making, including those with legal directives, such as (in the UK) Lasting Power of Attorney.

Box 4.8 Improving patient experience through enhanced partnership working

Bedfordshire's Partnership for Excellence in Palliative Support (PEPS)

Bedfordshire's Partnership for Excellence in Palliative Support (PEPS) pilot is helping to integrate all end of life care services in the area. It is based on a 'memorandum of understanding' between 15 local organisations and a central electronic register to which all individuals sign up. Two-thirds of deaths of those on the register have taken place in their usual homes. Meanwhile, the number of home deaths in the area has risen and the number of hospital deaths has fallen. The service has proved popular with individuals and their families. District nurses have also been reassured. They know now that if they need more support they can refer an individual to the palliative support worker who can sit with them through the dying phase if needed.

Inter-operability

In the piloting and testing of EPaCCS, it became apparent that for the system to be robust it is vital to have an agreed standard for the information to be collected, held and used. Specific information systems such as ones for end of life care have to fit with existing IT strategies and procedures within an organisation. Since end of life care covers diverse organisations and agencies, the likelihood of all sharing the same system are remote. Therefore the challenge is to find ways of enabling different systems to 'talk' to each other.

In the UK, the end of life care coordination national information standard (ISB 1580) specifies the core record content to be held on electronic end of life care coordination systems. By providing a standardised data set, the standard facilitates consistent recording of key information by health and social care agencies. It also supports safe and effective management and sharing of information with the consent of the individual and, importantly, it supports transfer of information between different IT systems.

Box 4.9 Improving inter-agency communication across multiple systems

Coordinate My Care – London

Coordinate My Care (CMC) is an integrated model of care, underpinned by IT, that has been rolled out across London. The service aims to provide better coordinated services by improving communications between hospital and community teams, including out-of-hours providers, NHS emergency services and the London Ambulance Service. The new system means any trained professional in the acute or community sector can set up a CMC record for any individual, regardless of diagnosis, who is identified as being in the last year of life. Each individual gives consent for a CMC record and this electronic record reflects ongoing end of life care discussions and advance care plans so that all care providers are kept up to date. The CMC record can be accessed 24/7 through a central password-protected secure internet connection used by the NHS. This allows professionals access only to that information which is relevant to them and their geographical areas of work. The system is being implemented across Sutton and Merton, Richmond, Twickenham, Croydon and Hillingdon healthcare areas. Over 2000 people are now on the register. A total of 429 people have died while on CMC, of whom 80 per cent achieved their preferred place of death and only 24 per cent died in hospital. More than half (51%) died in their usual place of residence, 12 per cent in hospice and 13 per cent in other locations.

Specialised care pathways

The needs of some groups of people are so complex and overlapping that coordination between care providers is vital but also extremely challenging. Skilbeck and Payne (2005) touch on the general principles and challenges of specialist palliative care services. They claim that current models of specialist palliative care may not necessarily be the most effective for addressing complex cases among non-cancer patients and strongly urge the development of new models of working. A classic pattern for non-cancer patients is that they may initially require services from only one branch of health and social care services but as their needs intensify other services are brought into play. People with dementia, for example, may attend a Memory Clinic for some years before they (and their carers) begin to require a range of increasingly intensive social care supports and in the final stages a range of medical treatments as well. Similarly, stable chronic heart failure may be effectively managed for some time before the person's condition becomes severe and palliative care is eventually required (National End of Life Care Programme/NHS Improvement 2010). The needs of such people may be best served by a dedicated integrated care pathway.

☞   STOP AND THINK!

What do you see as the advantages or disadvantages of specialist end of life care pathways?

Box 4.10 An end of life care pathway for people with dementia

A multidisciplinary working group in Hull and the East Riding of Yorkshire in the north of England has developed an integrated end of life care pathway for people with dementia and their carers in the area. It involves professionals from a range of statutory organisations as well as voluntary and independent organisations.

The Integrated Care Pathway outlines what actions need to happen to make the ideal journey a reality, who needs to be involved and what training is currently available. It also highlights the current gaps during different stages of the dementia journey.

The process, which is already benefiting people with dementia and their carers, has shown that many services are already in place, says the group, but prior to the pathway being established, there was a lack of awareness of one another's roles. The pathway has enhanced communication and coordination.

Conclusion

Good communication underpins all aspects of coordinated, integrated and seamless end of life care. Communication needs to be across professionals, organisations and agencies, but most importantly with individuals and their families so that their wishes and preferences can be met where clinically viable. Sharing of information about an individual to enable services to work together must be with the individual's consent and this is at the heart of achieving a successful, coordinated experience of care. We have seen that using electronic systems with agreed standardised information produces benefits for the individual and the organisation. Identifying a key worker or main coordinator who is known to all organisations and to the person and their family can be crucial to the provision of round-the-clock advice, care and support when needed.

However, underpinning all the strategies, tools and mechanisms for achieving coordinated end of life care must be the commitment from all organisations and agencies to work together across boundaries in the best interests of the person at the end of life.

Further reading

National End of Life Care Programme (2013) 'The Route to Success series.' Available at www. nhsiq.nhs.uk/resource-search/publications. aspx?pb=3841&rpp=5&sortby=Latest, accessed 25 September 2013.

National End of Life Care Programme (2012) 'Making the case for change – Electronic Palliative Care Co-ordination Systems.' Available at www.nhsiq.nhs. uk/resource-search/publications/eolc-epaccs-case-for-change.aspx, accessed 25 September 2013.

'The Gold Standards Framework Examples of Good Practice Resource Guide' (2006) Available at www.goldstandardsframework.org.uk/ Resources/Gold%20Standards%20Framework/Test%20Content/ ExamplesOfGoodPracticeResourceGuideJustInCaseBoxes.pdf, accessed 31 October 2013.

CHAPTER 5

Delivery of High Quality Care in Different Settings

Introduction

> It was worth getting her back home for that last month because if she'd died in hospital I'd never have forgiven myself. But you need all those things in place – support, friends, family, everything. (Former carer, quoted in National End of Life Care Programme 2010c)

Delivery of high quality services in all settings constitutes the fourth step in the end of life care pathway. There comes a point for many people where they may need end of life services in a number of care settings or require integrated care in one setting. Thus, they and their families/carers may need access to a complex combination of different services across a number of different settings. These settings can include hospital, community, care home, sheltered/extra care housing or hospices and on some occasions end of life care will also be needed in other locations such as prisons and hostels for the homeless. The particular needs of those with reduced capability for decision making also need to be considered, such as people with dementia or those with severe learning disabilities and mental health issues. Irrespective of who the person is, where they are and whether this is a place of their choosing, the same principles and standards of good end of life care apply:

> [People at the end of life] should receive the same high quality of care irrespective of the setting. People should have access to tailored information, specialist palliative care advice and spiritual care within a dignified environment, wherever that may be. (National End of Life Care Programme website)

Whilst technically not a service, continued access to local community support, such as contact with neighbours, membership of social clubs and societies and local church or faith communities, will also be important and add to the quality of experience for the individual and their families/carers.

In England end of life care has benefitted from its status as one of the Department of Health's Quality, Innovation, Productivity and Prevention (QIPP) national work streams since 2010, with an aim to improve the proportion of people who die in their usual place of residence, whether this is an individual's own home or a care home and to reverse observed trends towards institutional dying that have been reported in Britain and other developed world regions.

Recent work by Gomes *et al.* (2012a) shows that Britain is no longer part of the group of world regions such as Italy, Greece, Japan and Taiwan with trends towards greater institutionalisation of dying. They suggest that from 2004 onwards, it became more common for people in England and Wales to die at home, similar to the trend in the USA and Canada, and that this trend was sustained in the following seven years they examined. These changes were not brought about by differing data collection methodology or changes in the demographics of those dying, both of which could offer an explanation for the rise in home deaths, and imply that the trend reversal is real. In fact, with an ageing of the population, and a history of older people being less likely to die at home, one would have expected influences exerted in the other direction. They conclude that this indicates that within England the Department of Health's policy to improve end of life care services has had a sustainable impact.

☞   STOP AND THINK!

What is the relationship between preferred place of death and quality of services?

Defining quality

The US Institute of Medicine defines healthcare quality as:

> [t]he extent to which health services provided to individuals
> and patient populations improve desired health outcomes.
> The care should be based on the strongest clinical evidence
> and provided in a technically and culturally competent
> manner with good communication and shared decision
> making. Total quality is best defined as an attitude, an
> orientation that permeates an entire organisation, and
> the way in which that organisation performs its internal
> and external business. People who work in organisations
> dedicated to the concept of total quality constantly strive
> for excellence and continuous quality improvement in all
> that they do. (Pelletier and Beaudin 2008)

Quality in relation to end of life care can be defined in two ways. First there is the perception of receiving a quality care experience by the individual and their families/carers. This may be better expressed as measuring the satisfaction levels experienced by individuals and their families and be better understood when looking at this aspect of quality. Dy *et al.* (2008) completed a review of the literature to better understand the concept of satisfaction with end of life and palliative care. The review identified 21 relevant qualitative studies and was able to classify seven domains with a number of common themes. Although different studies defined the domains somewhat differently, there was general agreement on major areas of importance and most themes were identified in more than one study. This work is suggested as further reading at the end of the chapter.

This element of identifying quality will always be subjective, as it will be based on the views and experiences mainly of the bereaved, at a time of personal emotion, stress and upset. However, evidence-based methodologies are starting to be used, such as the VOICES survey in England, and will be discussed later in the chapter. Quality in England is also defined as the ability to deliver services that meet national measures based on the National Institute for Health and Care Excellence (NICE) quality standard for end of life care (NICE 2011), which can also provide information for assessments by the Care Quality Commission.

Quality of care in different settings

As the number of deaths within hospital settings decreases it becomes more urgent to examine the quality of end of life care across other settings, as up to now there has been little evidence that individuals who die outside of hospital, and their relatives, experience better quality care than those who die in hospitals, hospices or nursing homes.

Gomes *et al.* (2012b) reported on a cross-national survey undertaken to examine preferences for place of death for people facing advanced cancer. The areas covered were England, Flanders, Germany, Italy, the Netherlands, Portugal and Spain. The study found that 51 per cent in Portugal and 84 per cent in the Netherlands would prefer to die at home. These variations could not be explained by differences in age and gender distributions, but it is suggested that they could relate to the quality of local end of life care provision and macro social, economic and cultural factors. For example, the Portuguese findings may reflect concerns with the limited availability of home care and resources in the community, combined with a strong culture of traditional values leading to higher levels of respect for authority and the need to feel safe within institutions. This could explain why Portugal has the highest percentage of hospice/palliative care unit preferences and the third highest for hospital. By contrast, the higher preference for home deaths in the Netherlands may reflect the availability of home care, good economic circumstances and a culture where secular-rational and self-expression values are amongst the highest in the world.

The first VOICES survey (Department of Health 2012c) of bereaved people undertaken in England in 2010/11 showed over 50 per cent of respondents rating the quality of care in hospices, care homes and home settings as 'outstanding/excellent', compared with only 32 per cent in hospitals. This was the first very large-scale survey assessing the quality of support and care given to people approaching end of life in England and to their relatives and friends, and the feasibility of this approach has now been demonstrated. The approach was based on research by Addington-Hall and McCarthy (1995) and asked bereaved relatives about their perceptions of care given to recently deceased individuals. The approach is now well established and has proven valid in relation to evaluation of services. Further references to support this methodology can be found within the VOICES report.

Three findings are of particular significance. First, the overall quality of care across all settings was higher for cancer deaths, for deaths occurring in hospices and for younger deaths (under 65 years), although these three groups strongly overlap. The ratings of outstanding and excellent were lowest for patients who died in hospital. This pattern was confirmed by the quality of care questions that related specifically to each care setting, irrespective of where the patient died. Hospital doctors and nurses continued to be rated lowest for excellent quality of care and hospices were rated highest. Second, this survey highlighted significant differences in quality of care according to the age of the patient at death, cause of death and place of death. It is, of course, important to note that age at death, cause of death and place of death are interrelated. For example, 92 per cent of hospice deaths are due to cancer and 83 per cent of care home deaths were in those aged 80 years or older at death. Two-thirds of cardiovascular deaths and deaths due to other causes were in the 80 years and older group while two-thirds of cancer deaths are in the under-80 age group. In the future, with aggregated years of data, combined groups of cause and place of death can be compared. Third, the quality of care for patients where dementia was mentioned on the death certificate was generally rated of a similar standard to those without. For GPs and care homes, positive ratings of care were somewhat higher for patients with dementia than without but the opposite was true for hospital doctors and nurses. Three-quarters of responses reported GPs treated their patients with dignity and respect all of the time and that this did not differ between patients with or without dementia. For care homes, such ratings were slightly higher for people with dementia than without. Again, respondents were less likely to state that dignity and respect were shown all the time by hospital staff.

The VOICES report concluded that the survey had demonstrated that some patients receive high quality care, irrespective of age, cause of death or care setting. However, it has also revealed wide differences among patient groups and among care settings. The survey will be used as a baseline against which to measure progress on improving end of life care at both the national and local levels; a second VOICES survey was undertaken in 2012 reporting in 2013.

Many research projects reflect that most people say they want to die at home (Gomes *et al.* 2012b). However, this preference often changes as their disease trajectory progresses and whilst some reflect that their preferred place of care is at their normal place of residence they ultimately decide that they want to die either in hospital or in a hospice. Gerrard *et al.* (2010), for example, show through their study that place of care and place of death often become confused in initial discussions with individuals and whilst home is the most common preferred place of care this does not necessarily remain the preferred place to die.

In December 2012 the Department of Health in England published *Liberating the NHS: No decision about me, without me*, the government's response to a consultation that showed a commitment to introducing the right to choose to die at home (Department of Health 2012a). However, it must be acknowledged that providing choice does not necessarily lead to a quality experience. In reality, enabling individuals to have a choice will only be successful if there are end of life care services across settings and sectors that can provide high-quality options. In addition, the options open to an individual have to be balanced with clinical need, and realistically some individuals will not be able to have their preferences met if the care required cannot be safely delivered outside of a hospital setting. Munday, Dale and Murray (2007) suggest that for these choices to be meaningful there must be two or more high-quality options available that, in terms of dying, include home, hospice, hospital and nursing home.

☞   STOP AND THINK!

What factors do you have to consider when balancing choice against clinical need?

Socioeconomic factors also have an influence. For example, in more rural settings the proportion of individuals dying at home used to be greater that in more urban areas, especially in urban deprived areas. However, rural settings are progressively becoming places of high social mobility, with younger generations moving toward urban settings, potentially leaving those older people coping with both frailty and illness unable to rely on home care provided by family networks at the end of their lives (Surbone 2011). In her paper Surbone also suggests that cultural differences play a major role in shaping attitudes to end of life care matters including whether, when and how palliative services are provided. She suggests that the connection of religious and cultural variables to socioeconomic and socio-political factors in diverse countries and local contexts is insufficiently understood. She states that it will be crucial to systematically study all the variables that shape people's perspectives on health, illness, suffering and death and, consequently, their attitudes towards practices of and access to palliative and end of life care.

Surbone concludes that to offer satisfactory options to all individuals we must appreciate the cultural beliefs and values and religious traditions of different ethnic and cultural groups and integrate them into the design and implementation of high-quality palliative and end of life care services within each local context.

☞   STOP AND THINK!

How do you go about designing a service that takes account of religious and cultural variables?

Challenges

Drawing on wide-ranging experiences from end of life and palliative care practitioners, some common challenges emerge that are faced by those seeking to improve the quality of end of life care services across settings:

- Families are more mobile and dispersed than in the past, meaning that many older, ill and frail individuals are dependent on help from external agencies or that they have to be admitted to hospitals or care homes.

- Lack of integrated services – integrated end of life care across agencies and sectors provides a seamless service for individuals and their families, yet the various health, social care and voluntary agencies each have different funding levels and mechanisms and may have different priorities.

- Timely access to services – this links back to integrated seamless care and can be a small thing such as ensuring a hospital bed is available to be moved into a person's home for when they are discharged.

- Workforce culture change – for example, regarding good end of life care as quality care, rather than perceiving death as a failure to cure.

- Managing organisational change in such a way as to preserve the often fragile relationships which facilitate integrated working.

- Cultural challenges and beliefs of the individual need to be taken into account and reflected in their care. On occasions some of these practices and rituals may be unfamiliar to professionals and others providing care.

What does good look like?

The following sections look at what good looks like from the points of view of the individual and their family and of the practitioners providing care.

What does good look like in end of life care? The view of the person at the end of life

This section explains what good looks like in end of life care from an individual and their family's/carer's perspective. Good has been taken to mean 'having received a high-quality care episode'; for many, this will include their previously recorded preferences around where they prefer to be cared for and where they wish to die having been honoured and implemented. The following case study highlights the interaction among an individual, their family and care staff, and shows how the inclusion of advance care planning can not only support the individual's wishes but also take the burden of decision making at the final stage of life away from the family at a time when the individual may not be able to express their wishes.

Box 5.1 A quality experience

Gerald was 89 years old when he died. His wife had died five years before. They had been married for 60 years and had a son, Nick, who lived nearby and a daughter, Kate, who lived in Canada. Gerald lived at home for a year after his wife died, but found the house and garden difficult to manage. When Kate visited in the summer of 2007 she was shocked at how frail and unkempt he had become and he reluctantly agreed to move into sheltered housing. He lived there for two more years but was prone to falling and was becoming increasingly confused. He was on medication for hypertension but otherwise had no significant health problems. Kate came home twice a year and Nick visited most days. In 2009 Kate came home and was again very concerned about her father. His memory was much worse and he was finding it difficult to look after himself. He had urinary incontinence.

Kate had discussions with her father's GP, who assessed Gerald. The GP could find no specific physical health problems but arranged for him have a full assessment and further tests. The GP arranged for the district nurse to visit Gerald and she organised continence pads and a urinal. Gerald's daughter extended her visit. She worried about going back to Canada and leaving him where he was.

Gerald was diagnosed with moderate Alzheimer's disease. He was prescribed various medications, which it became clear over the next few days he was unable to manage. A family discussion led to agreement with Gerald that he would move into a nursing home. As part of his admission to the home in 2009, he and his family were encouraged to write down his wishes and preferences for care, which were lodged with the home. Lasting Power of Attorney was made, giving Gerald's son the right to make decisions on his behalf. All agreed that should his condition become worse he should be allowed to die in the home – with no 'heroics'. Gerald remained in the home. He deteriorated gradually but was well cared for. In December 2010 his condition worsened; he had a urinary tract infection and the GP was called. When she saw him he was very poorly and she diagnosed septicaemia. Nick was contacted and he called his sister, who arranged to fly home. They again agreed that there should be no 'heroics'. Gerald died that evening – Nick was with him and Kate arrived the following day.

Nick was sorry that his sister had not been able to be with them when their father died. However, he was glad that he had been there and in speaking to the GP and the home staff had realised that if the nursing home had called an ambulance (and this had been talked about in those last few hours), it was likely that Gerald would have died on the way to hospital or in A and E, which he felt would have been awful and against Gerald's and the family's wishes. Nick said that his father was happy in the home and very well cared for – it had become his home. He felt that the end had come quickly – his father would not have wanted to die in hospital and he would not have wanted a lot of fruitless treatment. He did not even recognise his grandchildren any more. Nick thought that his father would have felt that his funeral was appropriate. Gerald was buried with his wife who had been the 'love of his life' for over 60 years.

What does good look like in end of life care – the view of practitioners

This section looks at a model of service delivery designed to help services facilitate the person and their family experiencing a 'good' death. Good has been taken to mean 'having received a high-quality care episode'.

Box 5.2 Quality across settings in a local area

In 2011 County Durham and Darlington NHS Foundation Trust appointed two Macmillan Discharge Facilitators in the acute setting – one based at University Hospital of North Durham, the other at Darlington Memorial Hospital. They support rapid discharge of patients at the end of life into their preferred place of care and the discharge of palliative patients with complex needs.

The main aims of the post holders were to:

- improve the skills of ward based nursing teams in discharging complex patients with palliative care needs

- increase the proportion of dying patients who are managed on the Liverpool End of Life Care Pathway

- increase the numbers of palliative care patients able to die in their preferred place of care and

- improve the quality of palliative care patient discharge with the aim of reducing re-admission rates.

Their appointment has had a definite impact in terms of supporting preferred place of care, timeliness of discharge and coordination of care. Part of their role also involves contact with community staff and carers, often a time-consuming and slow process when undertaken by ward-based nurses, and this also ensures a good handover.

The Macmillan Carers service within County Durham and Darlington Foundation Trust also provides high-quality personal care and emotional support to patients approaching the end of life. The team comprises 16 highly skilled Health Care Assistants, who have enhanced skills in communication, person centred holistic care and providing intensive support for patients who are dying (and their families). They work very closely with District Nurses and the local Macmillan team to support early discharges and prevent admissions and to support patients and families to remain in their preferred place of care. The higher-grade staff are also expected to undertake some teaching.

The service is flexible, responds very rapidly and provides both practical support and care for patients and families. Increasingly the team are working with the two Macmillan Discharge Facilitators in the two acute hospitals who ensure that patients with end of life care needs in hospital are rapidly discharged to their preferred place of care. The Macmillan Discharge Facilitators have been able to work with A and E, Medical Admissions and all wards to ensure patients approaching end of life receive timely and appropriate investigations and treatment in hospital. They are also able to mobilise resources to ensure safe and effective discharges, sometimes within hours of admission. The Macmillan Carers are able to respond quickly to their requests for support.

Feedback from patients' carers and staff about both services is excellent – with many comments about the high levels of professionalism, respect for dignity and the focus on compassionate care. Service activity is increasing and the service is likely to expand further to meet the needs of the whole locality.

Within the same area, hospices have introduced rapid response teams as a joint project with their local commissioner and Marie Curie to cover small geographic areas. These comprise a qualified nurse and a Health Care Assistant trained in Palliative Care. The service is available 24/7 and undertakes to respond within an hour and be available for phone support as well. The Hospice Consultant offers training to Out of

Hours teams and GP registrars; one of the aims is to increase their confidence to treat within the home or care home and avoid unnecessary admissions. The Macmillan Discharge Facilitators do not refer all discharges to the hospice; this should only be done for those requiring Specialist Palliative Care – others are better suited to a nursing home/care home, even if they need palliative care, as these have become the person's home. The hospices link with care homes so that any care home resident who cannot be settled by the rapid response team in the home has access to a hospice 'assessment bed' for 48 hours. When the patient is able to leave the hospice they can go home, or as an alternative one of the nursing homes has identified 'step down' beds for those not fully ready to return to their home. The quality of services in the locality has improved by ensuring that discharge services are better managed and community services can respond to increases in patients being cared for in their normal home with support from local hospices.

Source: National End of Life Care Programme 2011b

An integrated person-centred approach

The case studies both show how integrated person-centred end of life care underpins a quality care episode as perceived by individuals, their families and carers and the staff supporting them on the end of life pathway. The main factors that need to be in place to support the delivery of an integrated care service can be seen to be:

- recognition and acknowledgement that someone is approaching the end of life ('Would I be surprised if this person were to die within 12 months/six months/three months?')

- holistic assessment, care plan, advance care planning – incorporating patient preferences and review

- tailored information for patient/family/carer that may be both verbal and written

- care coordination – communication between professionals and key information available to all (e.g., Electronic Palliative Care Coordination systems)
- 24/7 community support, generalist-based but with access to specialist advice/input
- bereavement support for carers
- a trained and competent workforce that includes both specialist and generalists in health and social care. Core components of this training are:
  - communications skills
  - assessment/advance care planning
  - symptom management
  - knowledge of how to use an integrated dying care pathway (in England, following the 2013 Neuberger Review 'More Care, Less Pathway – A Review of the Liverpool Care Pathway', known dying care pathways will be replaced by individual end of life care plans)
- integrated health and social care commissioning
- clear metrics and monitoring against quality standards e.g., in England these would include Care Quality Commission standards, the NICE Quality Standard for End of Life Care, End of Life Care Quality Markers, Key Performance Indicators on Patient Reported Outcomes that utilise both qualitative and quantitative data, and user involvement
- strategic leadership that includes both clinical and management leaders at all levels of the organisation, from board level to caregivers.

☞ STOP AND THINK!

How would you apply these factors to a care setting you are familiar with? Would you need them all?

The NICE Quality Standard for End of Life Care

In England, the NICE quality standard defines clinical best practice within end of life care. Although a specific tool to promote best practice in England, it draws on international evidence and therefore reflects what is commonly regarded as representing quality. The standard and the resources to support implementation and monitoring can be adapted and used by other countries that may be developing their services or used for comparison purposes. The quality standard provides specific, concise quality statements, measures and audience descriptors to provide the public, health and social care professionals, commissioners and service providers with definitions of high-quality care. It covers all settings and services in which care is provided by health and social care staff to all adults approaching the end of life. This includes adults who die suddenly or after a very brief illness. The quality standard does not cover condition-specific management and care, clinical management of specific physical symptoms or emergency planning and mass casualty incidents. It sets out markers of high-quality care for:

- adults aged 18 years and older with advanced, progressive, incurable conditions

- adults who may die within 12 months

- those with life-threatening acute conditions.

It also covers support for the families and carers of people in these groups. The quality standard describes high quality care that, when delivered collectively, should contribute to improving the effectiveness, safety and experience of care for adults approaching the end of life and the experience of their families and carers. It aims to help service providers and professions enhance the quality of life for people with long-term conditions, ensure that people have a positive experience of (health) care and treat and care for people in a safe environment and protect them from avoidable (healthcare-related) harm.

The quality standard comprises 16 quality statements (see Box 5.3) which together reflect good practice that can be found in end of life care services in many countries; as such, it should not really be presenting anything new to service providers and professionals who are committed to improving the quality of the end of life care episode for individuals and their families. However, it provides a useful benchmark and monitor.

Box 5.3 The NICE quality statements

1. People approaching the end of life are identified in a timely way.

2. People approaching the end of life and their families and carers are communicated with, and offered information, in an accessible and sensitive way in response to their needs and preferences.

3. People approaching the end of life are offered comprehensive holistic assessments in response to their changing needs and preferences, with the opportunity to discuss, develop and review a personalised care plan for current and future support and treatment.

4. People approaching the end of life have their physical and specific psychological needs safely, effectively and appropriately met at any time of day or night, including access to medicines and equipment.

5. People approaching the end of life are offered timely personalised support for their social, practical and emotional needs, which is appropriate to their preferences and maximises independence and social participation for as long as possible.

6. People approaching the end of life are offered spiritual and religious support appropriate to their needs and preferences.

7. Families and carers of people approaching the end of life are offered comprehensive holistic assessments in response to their changing needs and preferences, and holistic support appropriate to their current needs and preferences.

8. People approaching the end of life receive consistent care that is coordinated effectively across all relevant settings and services at any time of day or night, and delivered by practitioners who are aware of the person's current medical condition, care plan and preferences.

9. People approaching the end of life who experience a crisis at any time of day or night receive prompt, safe and effective urgent care appropriate to their needs and preferences.

10. People approaching the end of life who may benefit from specialist palliative care are offered this care in a timely way appropriate to their needs and preferences, at any time of day or night.

11. People in the last days of life are identified in a timely way and have their care coordinated and delivered in accordance with their personalised care plan, including rapid access to holistic support, equipment and administration of medication.

12. The body of a person who has died is cared for in a culturally sensitive and dignified manner.

13. Families and carers of people who have died receive timely verification and certification of the death.

14. People closely affected by a death are communicated with in a sensitive way and are offered immediate and ongoing bereavement, emotional and spiritual support appropriate to their needs and preferences.

15. Health and social care workers have the knowledge, skills and attitudes necessary to be competent to provide high-quality care and support for people approaching the end of life and their families and carers.

16. Generalist and specialist services providing care for people approaching the end of life and their families and carers have a multidisciplinary workforce sufficient in number and skill mix to provide high-quality care and support.

It is not expected that each quality statement will apply to all groups. Similarly, some quality statements may need special consideration when applied to certain groups. For example, people with dementia may need to participate in advance care planning significantly earlier in the pathway than people with cancer. The 16 statements have aligned with them 37 measures against which progress can be tracked.

Disseminating and developing quality across settings

Since the 2008 End of Life Care Strategy for England was launched, two types of tool have proven particularly effective in supporting its implementation. They work in different ways. The first, a growing database of practical evidence, at national and regional levels, of service innovations that have led to improvements in the quality of end of life care experienced by individuals and families, has continuously informed service delivery improvements and policy development through annual reports made to Department of Health Ministers. Known as the National End of Life Care Intelligence Network (NEoLCIN), it continues to provide systematic analysis of general and disease populations and trends in care needs and health and social care service delivery. The dissemination of this evidence base is focused on actively encouraging the sharing of good practices, quality and effectiveness across all parts of the system.

The second type of tool is those intended to support the development of good practice at the front line. The End of Life Care Quality Assessment (ELQuA) tool is designed to support any organisation caring for people at the end of life . The tool enables the organisation to keep track of progress on its delivery of improvements on the 37 measures which accompany the 16 NICE quality statements. The tool works seamlessly across statutory health and social care services as well as across voluntary and independent sector providers. The collation and dissemination of good practice examples (some of which are quoted throughout this book) is an important activity. Of particular importance in disseminating good practice guidance has been the development of a series called 'The route to success in end of life care' created in collaboration with numerous partners, professional groups and people with personal experience of end of life care. Based on person-centred care and the end of life care pathway, the publications provide practical support and guidance following the six steps of the pathway for health and social care staff and the organisations within which they work.

The following paragraphs summarise the guides available in the series and draw out common issues highlighted when addressing the challenges of delivering quality across settings (Step 4 within the guides) and can aid further discussion and learning. Some of the series have also been developed to reflect good practice identified for a small number of care groups with special needs and for professional groups involved in delivering quality end of life care. They provide a valuable resource offering signposting to other related resources and research.

The Route to Success – Care Homes (June 2010)

Enabling residents to die in comfort and with dignity is a core function of care homes. With better coordinated services and more support to care homes from health and social care services, the quality of care they provide at the end of life should enable more residents to die within the care home if that is their preference rather than within hospital through an emergency admission episode a few days prior to death.

The Route to Success – Acute Hospitals (June 2010)

More than half of all deaths occur in hospital. (ONS data supplied by South West Public Health Observatory, www.swpho.nhs.uk/). It is important that those who do die in hospital have receive a quality experience, but improved discharge arrangements and better coordination with a range of community services need to support more people to die at home if that is their preferred choice. This RtS is supported by a 'how to' guide.

The Route to Success – Hostels and Homeless People (December 2010)

Homeless people are often overlooked and described as a hidden population. The complexity of life for homeless people is reflected in the complexities of providing them with end of life care. Often hostels cannot deliver the care required and it is especially important to have policies in place when a crisis occurs at a weekend or in the middle of the night so that the transition to a hospital is well coordinated and minimises stress for the individual.

The Route to Success – People with Learning Disabilities (February 2011)

A number of people with learning disabilities will be significantly younger than the general population of dying people and may have multiple long-term physical and psychological problems that may make their care and access to appropriate end of life care placements complex.

The Route to Success – Domiciliary Care (February 2011)

There are particular challenges in relation to those domiciliary care workers, often described as home carers, who support people to remain in their own home. Domiciliary workers are often overlooked when policies are developed and are often not engaged in service development, yet they are providing care for a significant proportion of people at the end of life. There needs to be acknowledgement that they are unique lone workers; to support this, the United Kingdom Homecare Association (2003) has produced guidance for lone workers.

The Route to Success – Occupational Therapy (June 2011)

It is recognised that occupational therapists work in a diversity of settings and that they will be involved in the delivery of end of life care in different ways and at different times. These include acute care, rehabilitation, hospices, social services and re-ablement services, community services, care homes, services for people with learning disabilities, day care and prisons. They support continued participation in activities that are important for the person. The specific intervention will depend on the specific activity but could involve assistance to remain at work or to maintain independence in self-care for as long as possible.

The Route to Success – Nursing (July 2011)

Nurses support high-quality end of life care by contributing to, reviewing and maintaining the care plan, alerting the wider multidisciplinary team and other professionals as necessary to changes, as well as ensuring that the individual has the appropriate equipment to meet their needs. (This means that nurses in the community or a care home setting must be aware of how to access specialist equipment.)

The Route to Success – Environments of Care (August 2011)

There is now a great deal of evidence about the critical importance to individuals, families and staff of the environment in which care is provided. It not only supports recovery but is an indicator of people's perception of the quality of care. However, until relatively recently there has been little investment in identifying the aspects of the environment that are especially important for those receiving palliative care, their relatives and the bereaved. This RtS identified a number of key environmental principles to help improve privacy and dignity for patients and relatives and to support the bereaved, whose memories live on once their loved one has died.

The Route to Success – Prisons (Sept 2011)

It is generally acknowledged that many prisoners have complex needs, mental health problems and/or learning disabilities. Often, these will also be compounded by complicated family relationships, poor education and, for some, revolving admissions to the criminal justice system. This RtS looks at the complex combination of services across settings that prisoners may need access to, in order to receive high-quality care. This includes safety issues: staff must be accountable for the safe custody of the prisoner and the safety of the whole prison environment. Clear security procedures must be in place within the prison for individuals, visitors and medical staff bringing in prescribed medication and undertaking assessment and review of the patient. Clear procedures for considering whether release is appropriate on compassionate grounds need to be in place and readily available.

The Route to Success – Ambulance Services (February 2012)

Individuals and carers may need access to a complex array of services across a number of different settings as they approach the end of life. Ambulance services, including patient transport services and emergency ambulance services, are often involved in conveying people among these settings. This includes transfer between care homes. Although such transfers are often planned in advance, they can be fraught with complexities. In the absence of consistent policies, protocols and procedures across organisations and settings, delays are commonplace, resulting in inconvenience and distress to the person and carer as well as inefficient use of resources.

The Route to Success – Lesbian, Gay, Bisexual and Transgender People (June 2012)

LGBT people and their families and carers should have access to high quality end of life care that takes account of their needs and preferences. The RtS aims to be a practical guide for people working with LGBT people and for LGBT people themselves, whether giving or receiving end of life care.

The Route to Success – Social Work (July 2012)

Social workers are educated and experienced in working with loss and grief, helping individuals to adjust to changed circumstances and changed abilities, assessing their changing needs and working in partnership with the service user and their family to develop a care plan that is centred on their unique set of circumstances and characteristics. Social work is underpinned by a value base that respects the dignity of each person and their right to make important decisions about their lives and advocates for those people who are vulnerable or marginalised. Hence social work is well placed to support people at all stages on the end of life care pathway.

End of Life Care in Extra Care Housing

Fewer people living in extra care housing move into institutional care than people living in the community in receipt of domiciliary care (Neale 2010). Although not part of the Route to Success series, a learning resource pack for housing, care and support staff called *End of Life Care in Extra Care Housing* (2012) has been published jointly by the National End of Life Care Programme and the Housing Learning and Improvement Network. Based on the end of life care pathway but adapted to reflect the extra care housing setting, the guide is intended to reflect the journey of a resident living in extra care housing towards the end of life. Extra care housing describes many forms of housing for older people, but usually comprises homey, purpose-built independent housing units that feature common spaces and facilities and flexible care services. For many residents their home in extra care housing will be their home for the rest of their life. The resource pack recommends that an introduction to some end of life care skills should be included in the induction programme for new staff and that staff should be given guidance around the following policies and codes of practice to become confident in delivering quality end of life care:

- understanding that dying at home is a realistic option

- knowing the boundaries around preparing and witnessing legal documents, such as a will and Lasting Power of Attorney applications

- regulation and recommendations around recording information in a resident's file

- providing care in an emergency

- what to do when a resident has no next of kin

- boundaries around arranging and attending funerals

- duty of confidentiality to deceased residents (the Data Protection Act does not apply to the deceased).

Enhancing the healing environment

There is growing awareness of the importance of the environment within health care and we have already touched on the Route to Success looking at good practice relating to the environments of care in the previous section. The King's Fund's Enhancing the Healing Environment (EHE) programme encourages and enables nurse-led teams to work in partnership with patients to improve the environment in which to deliver care.

The report 'Improving the patient experience – Environments for care at end of life' describes projects in 19 NHS trusts and one HM prison in the UK that took part in schemes to improve the environment of care at the end of life. Each of the case studies includes photographs of the original space that was chosen for improvement and of the finished project. The projects featured show that, even in the most uninspiring environment, it is possible to create welcoming and comfortable spaces that are fit for purpose, provide good value for money and can improve the quality of care and the patient experience. The significance of this can be far-reaching:

> 'I don't think it's simply an environment change... The bereavement suite is right at the heart of the hospital and can't be ignored. End of life now has a higher profile. That's what we wanted.' (p.17)

A number of themes run across these guidance documents that point the way forward in achieving consistently high quality across all settings in which a person at the end of life may be receiving care. These themes can be translated into some key questions that organisations and practitioners should ask themselves when developing end of life care services (Box 5.4).

Box 5.4 Achieving quality in end of life care – key questions

- Has a policy for the management of end of life care been developed within your organisation? For example, what should happen at weekends or out of hours in end of life situations?

- What processes are in place for referral to other care settings and can you ensure the transition is well coordinated and minimises distress for the individual?

- Can all staff access any internal or external ongoing training and support programmes for end of life care?

- Does the environment within the organisation offer privacy, dignity and respect for individuals and their families as end of life approaches?

- What systems are in place to monitor and evaluate the quality and delivery of end of life care?

- How do both the organisation and the practitioners handle feedback from the people in their care and their families? Are complaints dealt with speedily and with respect? Do you have a system for noting what is valued?

☞   STOP AND THINK

List the improvements you could make in a care setting that you are familiar with.

Conclusion

In summary, as death approaches, individuals may move between different settings for elements of their care; the right residential setting may also change over time. At this point on the pathway, there are three priorities:

- ensuring that the transition between different settings is managed so that the individual's quality of life is maintained

- ensuring that change is minimised where possible

- ensuring that care is high quality wherever the individual happens to be.

We have seen that challenges exist when trying to measure quality in end of life care services. Many aspects of good end of life care can be objectively measured but, overwhelmingly, for the individual and their family it is a subjective experience, where what may have been a good, or bad, experience for one person is experienced differently by someone else in similar circumstances. However, inroads have been made in trying to determine quality or satisfaction levels of the care episode by methodologies that are gaining evidence-based validity. We have also discussed that being able to die in the preferred place of care is being used as an indicator of a quality experience, although there is not a strong evidence base to show a correlation between the two. Much of the work being undertaken in developing good end of life services focuses on services outside of the hospital setting, as research shows that significantly high levels of people would prefer to die in their home or normal place of residence. In the future, we must be able to expect that dying at home will equate to a good end of life care experience.

We have discussed some of the actions needed for service improvement and identified some of the resources available to improve the quality of services, and we have also seen that socioeconomic, cultural factors and religious and spiritual traditions need to be taken into account when designing and undertaking service improvements. These all add to the perception of a quality experience and higher satisfaction levels for the individual and their families, as well as giving greater satisfaction to staff delivering the service by knowing they are supporting the individual in the most appropriate way. For the individual and their families to experience a seamless, quality care experience generating high levels of satisfaction, services need to be delivered through integrated person-centred end of life care between organisations and across sectors. This challenge for quality end of life care becomes particularly important as the person's needs intensify and become more complex as they progress through the final stages of life.

Further reading

National End of Life Care Programme (2013) 'The Route to Success series.' Available at www.nhsiq.nhs.uk/resource-search/publications.aspx?pb=3841&rpp=5&sortby=Latest, accessed 25 September 2013.

Dy, S.M. *et al.* (2008) 'A systematic review of satisfaction with care at the end of life.' *Journal of the American Geriatrics Society 56*, 1, 124–129.

Huggard, J. and Nichols, J. (2011) 'Case study: Emotional safety in the workplace: one hospice's response for effective support.' *International Journal of Palliative Nursing 17*, 12, 611–617.

Department of Health (2012) 'First national VOICES survey of bereaved people: Key findings report.' Available at www.gov.uk/government/uploads/system/uploads/attachment_data/file/156113/First-national-VOICES-survey-of-bereaved-people-key-findings-report-final.pdf, accessed 21 May 2013.

Lundström, S., Axelsson, B., Heedman, P. et al. (2012) 'Developing a national quality register in end-of-life care: the Swedish experience.' *Palliative Medicine* *26*, 4, 313–321.

National Institute for Health and Care Excellence (NICE) (2011) 'Quality standard for end of life care.' Available at http://publications.nice.org.uk/quality-standard-for-end-of-life-care-for-adults-qs13, accessed 21 May 2013.

CHAPTER 6

Care in the Last Days of Life

Introduction

> Throughout her short illness Melissa's care was exemplary.
> I would never have thought it possible that I would say
> my young 20-year-old daughter could have a 'good death'.
> How can the death of a person so young be good? But it can
> be, with a combination of care, compassion, communication
> and common sense, all of which were applied in Melissa's
> care. (Ian Leech, father of Mel)

Care at the end of life is one of the most important caring activities we
can be involved in. It is not only the sole opportunity we ever have to
ensure that a person leaves this world without distress but also shapes
an experience that resonates powerfully with those left behind (Sykes
2012, in Oliver 2012, p.158). The most powerful memories of all for
bereaved relatives and friends often arise from the last few days and
hours of the person's life. It is this, within the end of life pathway, that
is referred to as the 'dying phase'.

> The point comes when an individual enters the dying phase.
> It is vital that staff can recognise that this person is dying,
> so they can deliver the care that is needed. How someone
> dies remains a lasting memory for the individual's relatives,
> friends and the care staff involved. It is important that the
> person dying can be confident that any expressed wishes,
> preferences and choices will be reviewed and acted upon and
> that their families and carers will be supported throughout.
> (National End of Life Care Programme website)

This chapter will focus on care in the last few days of life and will build upon the previous chapters. Best practice when caring for someone at the end of life involves the implementation of the previous steps in the care pathway including conversations about end of life, assessing need and planning care, multi-agency response to care coordination and delivering quality across care settings. Planning for care in the last days and hours of life, and enabling a good death, requires a step-by-step approach as evidenced within the preceding chapters.

There are many aspects to consider when caring for someone in the last few days of life. The purpose of this chapter is to provide some insights as to the key aspects, and is not intended to be a 'cover all'. Consideration will initially be given to care settings and the importance of health and social care working together for the benefit of the individual and those important to them. This is followed by exploration of the notions of good death and being treated with dignity, recognition of the dying phase, care pathways and symptom management. Brief exploration is given to the notion of 'being there' both physically and psychologically. The final section of the chapter will explore the vital role of the caregivers and the importance of those working within palliative and end of life care supporting one another. Case studies are used throughout to highlight good practice examples and also to illustrate where practice could have been improved upon. The chapter is punctuated with Stop and Think questions as an aid to encourage reflection and learning for the reader.

For the purposes of this chapter, 'care in the last few days of life' will be defined as the phase in life during which death is imminent. For some, this may be a gradual process, and indeed follow a steady decline along a predictable disease trajectory; for others this may be a sudden event with relatively little warning.

Care settings and place of death

The focus of the National End of Life Care Strategy (Department of Health 2008a) is to improve care for people at the end of life and is inclusive of all diagnoses and care settings. Individuals die in many care settings including hospitals, homes, care homes, hospices, prisons and hostels. Whatever the place of death, it is essential that each individual care setting strives to facilitate a good death for the individual and those important to them. Care in different settings may raise varied challenges for the professionals and carers involved. Implementing each of the steps identified within the end of life care pathway, including conversations, assessment, care planning and review and coordination of care, will enable improvements in the delivery of end of life care.

Location has been highlighted as a continuous theme within the literature with regard to the key elements that constitute a good death. It has been identified through a variety of surveys that the majority of the population state that they would prefer to die at home (Dying Matters 2013). Indeed, one of the key aims of the End of Life Care (EoLC) strategy is to enable people to have more choice and control over their place of care, and also in their place of death. The preference for dying at home for many individuals is about having more choice and control over their illness and medical interventions (Gott *et al.* 2008). For others it is also about being in familiar surroundings and having loved ones close by. Provision of and access to community support is variable throughout the country and is dependent on which services are commissioned and the provision of the voluntary sector care. If an individual identifies that they wish to die at home, it is important that this discussion be reflected on with the family and/or those close friends who will undoubtedly be required to undertake the majority of the care.

It is essential that health and social care professionals do not assume that they know where an individual would prefer to die; this should be explored as part of advance care planning conversations and should be revisited in any re-assessment. As people approach the end of life their preferences as to where they would like to die may change, hence professionals must reassess and ensure that they are aware of any changes in an individual's wishes and preferences, and that these are taken into account and acted upon appropriately. This is not to say that if a person has specified home as where they would like to die and within a few hours of death is asking to be admitted to hospital, that one should automatically call emergency services. Rather, it is about taking the time to ascertain what has led to that change, whether that truly is the decision that they would like to take, and whether there is anything more that can be done to support their original choice to remain at home.

I was caring for a gentleman at home with COPD who regularly changed his mind as to where he would like to die. Home, hospital, hospice and care home were all discussed on various visits. Through discussion, the place was not important; it was the 'how' that was taking up a lot of thinking time. Through taking the time to revisit his preferences I was able to address some of his deep-seated fears. He died at home, peacefully, with the cat on the end of his bed. (District nurse)

The reality is that the majority of the population die within an acute hospital – approximately 60 per cent in the UK (Dying Matters 2013) – and although numbers of deaths within hospitals are decreasing, many people will continue to die in hospital, at least in the immediate future. As with all care settings, hospitals should continue to strive to make improvements for those within their care (National End of Life Care Programme 2010d). The same good practice principles apply in hospitals as in any other setting and the following case study demonstrates what can be achieved in a setting that is often thought to be a second-class option for good end of life care.

Box 6.1 A good death in hospital

Robert was a 39-year-old man who was diagnosed with Cholangio cancer. The initial referral was for symptom management; however, it became evident that he was approaching the end of his life. He was of the belief that he would recover, recommence chemotherapy and have months – maybe years – to live. He and his partner had planned to marry the month following his first meeting with his specialist palliative care nurse. What ensued were many difficult emotional conversations with him, his partner and wider family around the fact that he would not recommence chemotherapy and would also not live long enough to marry at their pre-arranged date. As a result of these conversations they were supported to bring the wedding forward and to consider Robert's place of care at the time of his death. Due to his unstable and complex symptoms as well as the fact that he had young children at home, the couple decided to stay in hospital where they had close relationships with nursing and medical staff. The outcome was that Robert had his 40th birthday on the ward and also his wedding. The wedding was beautiful. It was held on the busy acute surgical ward at 11 o'clock on a Saturday morning. The registrar came in at short notice and nursing and medical staff came in on their days off to decorate the ward and support the whole family. Local businesses supplied wedding décor such as balloons and chair covers and the hospital trust provided a buffet and drinks. A camera was provided by one of the doctors for photographs to be taken throughout the whole day, leaving wonderful memories for all of them. Sadly, Robert died the following Saturday, 11 weeks after diagnosis. The family said that they felt 'at home,' supported and prepared.

Source: Carolyn Wills, clinical nurse specialist, hospital specialist palliative care team

---

☛ STOP AND THINK

What could you as an individual, or the organisation within which you work, do differently to ensure that individuals and those important to them experience good end of life care?

Working together

One of the main drivers, and indeed challenges, within health and social care services is that of working together for the benefit of the individual. Current policy is driven by and focuses on integration of care and collaboration. All too often, however, and specifically when staff are under stress, working in 'silos' becomes the norm, collaboration sometimes not extending beyond the immediate team.

There are essentially two issues here: first, lack of communication and interdisciplinary working within a particular specialism among professionals of different groupings (nurses, physicians, etc); and second, a lack of interdisciplinary working across specialisms (oncology and palliative care, for example).

Curtis and Shannon (2006) explore the impact of nurse–physician communication on quality of care at end of life in the ICU. The authors claim that physician and nursing cultures tend to be organised as silos with the result that, despite working alongside one another to achieve the same goal, physicians and nurses rarely interact and have a limited understanding of each other's work. Interdisciplinary communication and collaboration is, according to the authors, rarely achieved within this environment. In fact, commenting on the US context, Connor *et al.* (2002) claim that interdisciplinarity, whilst essential within end of life care, is truly provided only within hospices. As such, the authors propose a range of potential solutions and interventions for improving interdisciplinary team working, including staff training in this area and re-worked payment structures. Nelson (2006) explores the silo effect of splitting healthcare into disciplines and specialities as a significant barrier that weakens quality end of life care in intensive care units. Selwyn (2008) also discusses the problematic division of specialist fields into silos, a division that runs counter to patients' experiences of illness and which results in 'adverse consequences' for both professionals and patients alike.

It is essential that health and social care professionals be aware of the roles and responsibilities each other can have when supporting individuals and those important to them. The following case study highlights the importance of good team working and what this can achieve for the individual.

Box 6.2 Working together to facilitate choice

Helen was a 73-year-old woman with a diagnosis of endometrial cancer. She was admitted to the acute hospital following a sudden deterioration in her condition. She was experiencing weight loss and vomiting and was diagnosed with intestinal obstruction. Helen was advised by her oncologist that she was not able to undertake any further disease-modifying treatment and that it was now important to focus on management of her symptoms and keep her comfortable. Helen was then referred to the hospital palliative care team who met with her to discuss her symptoms and care needs. It was quickly identified that Helen had a strong desire to return home, and to be cared for at home until she died. Helen had become so weak that she was now bed bound and was requiring a continuous subcutaneous infusion to manage her symptoms. The palliative care nurse involved the occupational therapy team to assist with ensuring all relevant equipment including a hospital bed was quickly delivered to Helen's home as her prognosis was poor and her condition rapidly deteriorating. The palliative care nurse arranged a meeting with Helen's family, the ward medical team, OT, and a member of the local district nursing team and discharge liaison to discuss discharge, which enabled care to be arranged in a timely manner. Helen was discharged home within two days of expressing her wishes, with a full package of care and the support of her local hospice team and Marie Curie night sitters. Helen's family were able to make arrangements to enable them to spend time with, and help care for, their mother whilst being supported by the District nursing and hospice team. Helen died at home three days later, in her preferred place, with her family around her.

Source: Susanne Bradley, end of life care
education and pathway facilitator

One group of staff who may not be routinely called upon in palliative care settings but whose skills particularly come into play in situations of conflict or complex family dynamics are social workers. As the Route to Success in end of life care for social work (National End of Life Care Programme 2012b) highlights, social workers' training in managing difficult situations and stressful emotions, their guiding principle of empowerment and working in partnership with the service user and their common role of negotiating among different service providers as well as different family members, equips them to respond to the often fraught and complex psycho-social problems that can arise when someone is dying. It is important that all available skills and resources be brought to bear on situations where care is falling short.

Box 6.3 The role of social work in a crisis

Paul, aged 75, was admitted to a surgical ward in a busy acute hospital for exploratory surgery, only to find that he had widespread disease. His condition deteriorated very quickly and it became clear that he was likely to die within days. The busy ward team were unable to provide adequate palliative care; Paul became withdrawn and his family were angry and distressed that he had not been correctly diagnosed earlier and vented their frustration upon the medical and nursing staff on the ward. Witnessing the escalating crisis, the social worker from the hospital's specialist palliative care team quickly intervened to help resolve it. Building on her existing working relationships, she was able to bypass the hospital's normal bed management system to get Paul transferred to a single room where he could be cared for in a more peaceful environment. She then worked with the palliative care consultant and ward nurses to ensure Paul's symptoms were managed and that he was as comfortable as possible. Once the immediate care crisis had been resolved, she then spent time with Paul and family members individually and helped them to work through their anger and to talk to one another. Family members felt that they had been listened to and that Paul himself was now being cared for as well as possible. This allowed the family to put aside their anger and to make the most of the remaining few days of his life.

Source: National End of Life Care Programme 2012b, p.33

☞   STOP AND THINK

Do you understand the roles of all professionals you have contact with? What can you do to enhance your understanding?

A good death

One of the key concepts to discuss when looking at the last few days of life is the notion of a 'good death' or 'dying well'. This has been explored within the literature for several decades. However, the profile of end of life care has grown in momentum and recognition and has been seen increasingly as a priority following the publication of Lord Darzi's Final Review (Department of Health 2008a) and the End of Life Care Strategy (Department of Health 2008a). Achieving a good death is now seen as both a social and political priority (Ellershaw *et al.* 2010). One of the key aspects from both the review and the strategy is the focus on choice and on ensuring that people are supported to die within the place of their choosing wherever possible.

What does good care at the end of life look like? What is important to people as they approach the end of life? Throughout the 1990s we see increasing attention to these complex questions. A significant marker was laid down in 1999 with the publication of 12 key principles set out by the Age Concern Debate of the Age Health and Care Study Group. Although of particular concern to older people whose dying had been marginalised with significant inequalities experienced in access to palliative care services (Holloway 2007) this statement comprehensively covers the range of issues applicable to every person's death.

Box 6. 4 Principles of the good death

1. To know when death is coming and to understand what can be expected.

2. To be able to retain control of what happens.

3. To be afforded dignity and privacy.

4. To have control over pain relief and other symptom control.

5. To have choice and control over where death occurs (at home or elsewhere).

6. To have access to information and expertise of whatever kind is necessary.

7. To have access to any spiritual or emotional support required.

8. To have access to hospice care in any location, not only in hospital.

9. To have control over who is present and who shares the end.

10. To be able to issue advance directives which ensure wishes are respected.

11. To have time to say goodbye, and control over other aspects of timing.

12. To be able to leave when it is time to go and not to have life prolonged pointlessly.

Source: Age Concern London 1999

☞ STOP AND THINK

What would a good death mean to you?

Four overarching themes which resonate cross culturally have been identified as pertaining to a good death:

- being treated as an individual, with dignity and respect

- being without pain and other symptoms

- being in familiar surroundings

- being in the company of close family and/or friends.

(National End of Life Care Strategy,
Department of Health 2008a, p.9)

Holloway (2007) highlights another aspect to this, namely 'dying in peace and with one's affairs in order' (Holloway 2007, p.100). It is important to note that these are overarching principles, and just as every person is an individual and every life lived is 'unique', so is each death as unique as that individual (Nuland 1995). Benz and Chand (2012, p.185) remind us that 'Dying may be universal, but each death is uniquely individual'.

A good death is a concept that is 'nebulous and fluid' (Allen *et al.* 2012) and health and social care workers must ascertain, through discussion, what is important to each individual within their care and the specific nuances that may be important to that person. Any specific aspects identified must be recorded within the care planning and shared (with the permission of the individual) with the relevant teams.

Reflecting on the first point, being treated as an individual with dignity and respect, one might ask *What is a 'respectful' death?* Faber *et al.* (2004) write that a respectful death is one that is supportive of the dying person, their families and health care professionals in the completion of the life cycle. There is a great deal of discussion in the literature focusing on dignity and respect. The year 2006 saw the launch in the UK of the Dignity in Care Campaign (Department of Health 2006b). To date there are 40,000 individuals and organisations who have signed up to promote and ensure that dignity and respect are core values within service delivery (Dignity in Care Network). Dignity champions work in health and social care and believe that being cared for with dignity is a human right and not an optional extra. There are 10 core values that services must embody to ensure that people's dignity is respected at all times.

Box 6.5 Core values of dignity in care

1. Have a zero tolerance of all forms of abuse.

2. Support people with the same respect you would want for yourself or a member of your family.

3. Treat each person as an individual by offering a personalised service.

4. Enable people to maintain the maximum possible level of independence, choice and control.

5. Listen and support people to express their needs and wants.

6. Respect people's right to privacy.

7. Ensure people feel able to complain without fear of retribution.

8. Engage with family members and carers as care partners.

9. Assist people to maintain confidence and a positive self-esteem.

10. Act to alleviate people's loneliness and isolation.

Source: Dignity in Care 2013

Dignity in care is an important aspect of all health and social delivery. It is about ensuring that all services are truly focused on the care of the individual; this is important at all times, but one could argue that this is never more vital than when caring for people at the end of their life. Dignity in care should be a core value for all, and its impact never underestimated.

☛ STOP AND THINK!

Is there more that you and/or your organisation could be doing to promote dignity in care?

Recognition of the dying phase

Recognition of when death is approaching is an important aspect to ensuring that care delivery is responsive to the needs of the individual, and to supporting the person to be cared for in their preferred place of care and to die in the place of their choosing. Only by recognising and diagnosing that death is imminent can the optimal symptom management be provided and futile invasive treatments avoided. This in itself can cause challenges, as the cumulative effect of advances both in medicine and technology has meant that at times individuals and indeed physicians believe that death can be avoided (Angus *et al.* 2004). Those challenges can impact on both professionals and individuals alike.

> I've been a nurse for 30 years, 25 of which have been focused on quality end of life care. I have seen more 'suffering' today than I did 25 years ago. Our technology has surpassed our humanity. (Ferrell 2006, p.927)

By recognising and diagnosing that someone is dying, the focus of care can be around enabling a good death. However, diagnosing dying is not always straightforward and there can be challenges to identifying when an individual is approaching the end of life, particularly for those with long-term conditions or neurological disease, and for frail older people and those with co-morbidities. It should be noted that it is important not to give too much weight to prognostication; rather, the focus should be on the preceding steps of the care pathway (as outlined in Chapter 1) in relation to assessment and care planning, ensuring that everything is in place 'just in case', and that the workforce can react appropriately and in a timely manner to the needs of the individual. Additionally it is about looking at the person him- or herself and noticing the changes that may be occurring. This ability 'to know' may come through many years of experience and intuitive practice and it is important that junior staff be able to work alongside senior practitioners as they hone their own expertise.

Recognition of the dying phase is also important to ensure that effective, open and honest communication is fostered with the individual and those important to them. It provides those final opportunities to say some of the words that may have been unspoken. For many it is the final opportunity to tell someone that they are loved and to say goodbye, and for some to put past grievances behind them. This is one of the reasons why it is so important that the person who is dying and their families be told the truth; the alternative is that we are at risk of preventing and denying those final important moments.

> I vividly recall one family who knew that George was dying. Each of the grandchildren aged 7 to 17 were asked if they would like to go and tell him something special. Each grandchild sat on his bed, gave him a cuddle and whispered something in his ear; each child had a cuddle in return and something special whispered back. Precious moments. George died the next day. (District Nurse and carer for George)

As highlighted in Chapter 2, professionals have an ethical responsibility to give the person who is dying and those important to them every opportunity to use the time remaining in the way that is most important to them. Achieving quality care at the end of life is a highly individual process and should be achieved through shared decision making, clear communication and the timely sharing of information. But as George Bernard Shaw reminded us, 'The single biggest problem in communication is the illusion that it has taken place' (BookBrowse 2013).

Box 6.6 Understanding that death is imminent

My Mum was being cared for in hospital. She had been diagnosed with multiple myeloma two years previously. The consultant was wonderful and communicated openly and honestly with my Mum at the outset. He told her, 'Mary, I can't cure you…but I can make you feel much better than you do today.' From diagnosis my Mum received excellent care from both the hospital and the community services. She had several admissions to hospital for symptom management, including several blood transfusions. On one particular admission she seemed to me to be rather sleepy, was very content just not engaging very much. I had been due to go away for a long weekend with some of my nursing colleagues;

however, I decided to stay with Mum. My closest and dearest friend chose not to go away either, and journeyed 350 miles to spend some time with me and Mum. When Sam arrived, I was at the hospital with Mum; she popped in, gave us both a hug, and promptly left the room. I became aware that she was crying out in the corridor, very faint sobs. I left my Mum's side feeling rather confused and went to give her a hug. When I asked what the tears were for, she looked at me and said, 'I had no idea that your Mum is this poorly... She is dying.' Looking back, Sam could see what I, as Mary's daughter could not see. I thought Mum had been admitted for another transfusion. For all the wonderful care my Mum had received, no one had actually told me that she was dying. She died the following day on Mothering Sunday – thanks to Sam I had the opportunity to say goodbye and tell her how much I loved her and was going to miss her.

Source: Daughter of Mary and nurse

Dying care pathways

The origins of integrated care pathway models were within the engineering and manufacturing industry with the intention of ensuring consistency and decreasing costs whilst maintaining quality (Watts 2012). This approach was initially introduced within healthcare in the early 1980s in Boston, Massachusetts and was based upon collaboration and a multidisciplinary approach, enabling nurses to manage the care in a more 'dynamic' manner (Ellershaw *et al.* 2001). Within the UK, the driver behind the Integrated Care Pathway was to transfer the ideals of hospice care into other care settings (Ellershaw *et al.* 1997). The Liverpool Care Pathway for the dying patient (LCP) was developed at the Marie Curie Institute Liverpool and was one of the tools recommended with the National End of Life Care Strategy (Department of Health 2008a).

The LCP is a multidisciplinary tool comprising three discrete sections that focus on the dying phase; these are initial assessment, continuing assessment and care after death. The pathway promotes holistic care of the individual and those important to them. Additionally, the LCP provides a clear methodology for measuring symptom control and developing guidelines and can be used as part of a continuous audit and education program (Ellershaw *et al.* 2001). It is important to note that, as with any pathway, the level at which it is used and implemented is dependent on the skills and understanding of the professionals involved; communication is once again key both with the individual and those important to them and also within the multidisciplinary team.

In 2013 the Department of Health in England commissioned an independent review of the Liverpool Care Pathway which was led by Baroness Julia Neuberger and published in July 2013: 'More Care, Less Pathway – A Review of the Liverpool Care Pathway'. Baroness Neuberger said:

> There is no doubt that, in the right hands, the Liverpool Care Pathway supports people to experience high quality and compassionate care in the last hours and days of their life. But evidence given to the review has revealed too many serious cases of unacceptable care where the LCP has been incorrectly implemented.

As a response to the review, an end of life care plan will replace dying care pathways for individuals in England and be supported by improved good practice and condition-specific guidance as well as additional training for professional and care staff.

Symptom management

Effective management of an individual's symptoms at the end of life is one of the key elements to achieving a good death. Holistic care of the individual ensures that all aspects of symptom management are addressed including the physical, psychological and spiritual. Each individual will experience different symptoms, and different nuances of those symptoms. Broadly speaking, Ellershaw *et al.* (2010) identify four main physical symptoms associated with the terminal phase, namely pain, nausea, sickness and respiratory tract secretions. Other symptoms may include fatigue, anxiety and constipation (Hunwick *et al.* 2010). However, to ensure optimal symptom management and alleviate suffering, it is essential that the issues of psychological distress are also attended to (Kelly *et al.* 2006), and, additionally, that spiritual aspects are encompassed within the assessment process:

> Death is not primarily a medical event. Death is a personal, relational, and spiritual event, yet the majority of professional effort is concerned with the medical aspects of the end of life, often to the neglect of the more pertinent issues facing the dying and their families. (Watson 2010, p.46)

One of the key aspects to achieving optimal symptom management is ensuring that the appropriate medication is available at the right time. Pain medication is available in a variety of administration methods, for example, oral, injectable or suppository. Good practice is to ensure that anticipatory prescribing has taken place, and that medication to alleviate any 'anticipated' symptoms is available within the individual care setting.

Most symptoms can be effectively managed within generalist care. It is, however, of paramount importance that community healthcare professionals be aware of local referral pathways, and in particular of how to access specialist palliative care support. The latter should be available to all individuals at the end of life, not just those with a cancer diagnosis, therefore ensuring equitability of services for all. Specialist palliative care teams work within all care settings to provide psychological and symptom support. A referral to these services may be needed when the symptoms (psychological or physiological) exceed the knowledge of the generalists involved. Specialist palliative care services are available to support both the individual and those important to them and to offer support and guidance to generalist staff.

Box 6.7 Quality care through teamwork

From the moment we were told her non-Hodgkin lymphoma was incurable, a clear plan was set out and was discussed with all those who were and would be involved in her care, including our family. On hearing the news, Melissa explained

that her two wishes were that she wanted to be with her family
and she wanted to die at home. From that moment, all efforts
were concentrated on making that happen. The staff who
had been caring for Melissa in hospital communicated with
the district nurses and us. They spoke with consultants and
staff at our local hospital where Mel had first been diagnosed
and arranged oxygen deliveries to our home. With Melissa at
home and settled downstairs, we were visited by our district
nurse, who knew all about Mel, not just as a patient, but as
a person. She used that knowledge to instil confidence and
build a strong trust between herself and Melissa. Her first
question to Mel was, 'What can I do to make you more
comfortable?' As a family we knew immediately that here was
someone we could trust. The GP visited the following day
and, again, reaffirmed our trust that we were in the hands of a
great team. Our district nurse arranged a local hospice nurse
from St. Giles Hospice to visit who helped with ensuring
Melissa had all the right medication in place. It was teamwork
at its very best. Everyone knew each other's role and at every
turn we, as a family, were consulted. As Melissa's condition
deteriorated she was placed on the Liverpool Care Pathway
and this ensured the high-level of quality care continued.
Nothing was done and no decisions [were] made without Mel
and the family being involved. When the time came to discuss
resuscitation, this was done in a timely and compassionate
manner by our GP. Mel's initial reaction was that she wanted
to be resuscitated, but within eight days, her condition had
deteriorated and she changed her mind. This taught me the
importance of talking about dying and the need, as hard as it
may be, to have these difficult conversations.

Good end of life care should be the right of everyone and
there was no aspect of Melissa's care that was age specific; her
level of care could have been given to anyone of any age. All
it took was care, compassion, common sense and, probably
most important of all, good communication.

Source: Ian Leech, Mel's Dad;
family website: www.mad4mel.co.uk

Being there

Effective communication throughout the care pathway is pivotal to ensuring that high-quality care is delivered and that care remains in line with, and focuses on, the wishes and preferences of the individual. Communication is the key thread that runs throughout each step of the end of life care pathway; it is the one single key that opens all the locks. Communication impacts on every minute aspect of care; Buckman (2000) highlighted that without effective communication 'effective symptom management is virtually impossible'.

One of the most important aspects of good communication is listening actively and being present in mind, body and soul. In the words of the Greek Philosopher Epictetus, 'We have two ears and one mouth, so may listen more and talk less.' Listening to the individual and those important to them is an essential aspect of end of life care. What is important is physically being present, listening, taking an interest; it is not always about having to actively 'do something'. The importance of end of life conversations was covered in Chapter 2 and, with that in mind, this section is brief and relates to the notion of 'being there' and being present in the moment: 'The greatest gift that we can offer anyone is our true presence' (Thich Nhat Hanh (2005) in Johns 2006).

In a systematic literature review of spiritual care at the end of life, Holloway *et al.* (2011) found that practitioners identified 'being there' and offering 'a compassionate presence' as significant elements in spiritual care. It is important to remember the vital role of non-verbal communication. Non-verbal communication is about transmitting attitudes and beliefs through gestures, facial expressions and body language (Brooker 2002). A great deal can be expressed through non-verbal communication: a gentle touch, a look, or reaching out to hold someone's hand can be as effective as words and at times can be more powerful.

Box 6.8 The healing touch

Julie was a 47-year-old woman who was terminally ill with pancreatic cancer. She mentioned to her palliative care nurse that as she was becoming more unwell, the nurses seemed to be avoiding eye contact and the doctors stood at the end of her bed, whispered 'palliative' and moved on. She felt very lonely and isolated but was comforted by the gentle touch of a healthcare assistant. Julie said that single gentle touch on her arm conveyed so much; no words were needed, she felt empathy, comfort and warmth from that single gesture.

Source: Sonia Thompson, Palliative Care Specialist Nurse

Carers

Many people who choose to die at home will have input from a significant number of professionals including district nurses, general practitioners, social workers, specialist nurses and allied health professionals. However, the reality for most people who choose to die at home will be that they will require significant support and input from their family and/or those close to them. Indeed, for many caregivers, this may be first time that they have 'nursed' a loved one at home; and for many it may be the first time that they will have been with and supported someone in the dying phase. This is an experience that has a profound impact on any carer, one that may be a cherished memory or the source of ongoing distress: 'The experience of caring for loved ones as they approach death can be one of deep fulfilment or significant trauma' (Rabow *et al.* 2004).

Let us first consider two questions: What is a carer? And who are carers? The Carers Trust defines a carer as:

> ...someone of any age who provides unpaid support to family or friends who could not manage without this help. This could be caring for a relative, partner or friend who is

ill, frail, disabled or has mental health or substance misuse problems... Carers don't choose to become carers: it just happens and they have to get on with it... (Carers Trust 2012)

In order for people to remain at home, it is vital that health and social care professionals support the informal caregiver to enable them to fulfil their role. Without support and guidance, the burden of the caregiver may become too great. Thomas (2003) highlights that '[c]arer breakdown is THE key factor in prompting institutionalised care for dying patients' (Thomas 2003, p.239). It is important that health and social care workers ask the 'how are you?' question and take time to listen to the response and ascertain ways of providing the caregiver with support.

There have been several challenges identified for family caregivers including carer ill health, lack of skills to manage both symptoms and physical tasks, lack of support from health professionals, financial costs, stress from other family members and lack of time for self (Rabow *et al.* 2004; Hudson 2004). One of the key difficulties, perhaps, is how individuals manage the role of carer within the midst of life. Most are juggling ongoing family life and some are also in paid employment alongside the role of caregiving. Macmillan Cancer Support highlights the importance for carers to be able to live life in a way that is as close to normality as is possible (Macmillan Cancer Support 2012b); for many people there is something quite reassuring about routine. In the final phase of life, routines may change completely and it is helpful for professionals to remind and reassure carers that they need to take time for themselves, to rest and to ensure that they are nourished in terms of food and drink.

As highlighted, for many caregivers this may be the first time that they have cared for someone at home and therefore they will have limited knowledge of the physiological and psychological changes that may occur prior to death. The caregiver may not notice some of the subtle changes that may signify that death could be imminent. These changes should be brought to the caregiver's attention; for example, asking a simple question such as 'How do you think [the person's name] is today? Have you noticed any changes?' It is important that carers be aware of some of the changes that may occur so that they know what to expect, especially at a time when there may be no health or social care professionals present. The following are just some of the changes to highlight.

- The need for food and drink diminishes and this is a natural part of the dying process.

- The person may withdraw from interaction and become less interested in what is happening around them.

- The person may sleep more and may slip in and out of consciousness.

- S/he may no longer be able to swallow.

- The skin may become discoloured.

- Peripheries (e.g., feet, hands) become cold.

- Changes in breathing, which may become more laboured and noisy.

- The person may become restless and agitated.

By being aware of the changes above, the carer is less likely to panic and call the emergency services, which too often results in the person being admitted to hospital rather than being supported to die at home as they may have indicated was their wish. However, it is important that carers are aware of any action they can take to ease the person's dying.

It is also important that a conversation take place with the caregiver regarding what needs to be done just after the death in terms of who to contact (both in and out of hours). Families often think that they should 'do something' immediately. It is important to reassure the caregiver that if the person dies late at night or in the early hours, the choice is either to call the out-of-hours doctor service or, if they prefer, to wait until normal surgery hours and call their own GP. There is no right or wrong way and the choice should be made by the caregivers. Likewise, there is no immediate need to call the undertaker; families may choose instead to sit with their loved one for a few hours prior to making contact with funeral services.

> The district nurse was insistent that I should call the undertakers just after Mum had died – it was late at night, cold and raining, and we were emotionally and physically

> exhausted. We had already had a stranger come to 'certify' her death and I decided to leave that call until the morning. My Mum was able to leave our home in daylight in a dignified way. (Daughter and social worker)

For many, caring for a loved one at home can be deeply fulfilling, but some carers may not feel able to continue caring for their loved one in the last few days of life. Paddy (2011) argues that hospital should always be highlighted as an option, especially if the person becomes very unwell and agitated, and that admission to hospital followed by death should not be seen as a failure. This is an unnecessary burden of guilt for the caregiver when the person has died.

The role of the health and social care professionals is one of walking alongside the caregiver, providing information, guidance and reassurance; it is about being one step ahead at all times.

☞   STOP AND THINK!

How could carers be supported better within the organisation where you work?

Caring for each other

Working within palliative and end of life care can be deeply fulfilling, rewarding, challenging, painful, and even joyous on occasions. In order to be effective and care in a truly holistic manner, practitioners '...need to learn to embrace and survive intimacy rather than resist it because it's too painful at times' (Johns 2006, p.33). Contrary to what many believe, it is often the loss of caring that causes burnout, not the caring itself (Benner and Wrubel 1989 in Johns 2006). It should be recognised that there are times when communication can be a challenge for health and social care professionals when supporting individuals in the terminal phase. To enable practitioners to care at that 'intimate' level and to prevent burnout, it is essential that support mechanisms be in place within the workplace.

This support may be provided through clinical supervision and mentoring, or less formally through discussion with colleagues, or through such devices as the keeping of reflective journals. The busyness of practitioners' working days, the complexity of teams and lone working, particularly within the community, can present challenges in terms of connecting with colleagues. It is important that mechanisms be in place to ensure that practitioners feel supported and cared for within their workplace. Managers have a responsibility to ensure that their workers are cared for and valued and that time for reflection is regarded as essential, not as an optional luxury. Despite these challenges, when properly supported, working with families and individuals at the end of their life is hugely rewarding and many workers regard it as a privilege. As this hospital social worker commented, 'My work with people who are dying or bereaved brings me immense satisfaction. It represents the "purest" elements of my work' (Lloyd [Holloway] 1997, p.182).

☛   STOP AND THINK!

How could your team support one another more effectively?

Box 6.9 Being a palliative care nurse

I've nursed the dying for twenty-five years and it has never depressed me. Inevitably, there are many times I have shared and felt sadness along the way. I have learnt not to own that sadness, any more than we own the sadness we see on the news. Being a nurse isn't what I do, it's what I am. I choose to 'be there' to walk alongside, help if I can, comfort always and then walk away into my own life. A life with its own stresses and challenges, where I make mistakes and laugh as often as I can. I try 'not to sweat the little stuff'. The superficial and inconsequential fail to engage me. If I forget to put my make up on before I go out – who cares? My role has given me the freedom to care less about nonsense and more about the meaningful. Our knowledge, skills and insight matter;

we are 'the face' people talk to, the sponge that absorbs their feelings, helps them to 'makes sense of them' and leads them to a place of emotional safety. We are memory makers and pain relievers. I've laughed and cried when I shouldn't have. Worried when I couldn't change it, tried too hard and blamed myself too often. But, alongside all those patients I did care, really cared, and I grew, grew to be someone who does stop and smell the roses, will wear purple and is very proud to be a nurse. I'm just a nurse, and I wouldn't change a minute of it.

Source: Janet Dunphy, Clinical Nurse Specialist, Palliative Care, Kirkwood Hospice, Huddersfield

Conclusion

Care in the last few days of life encompasses many fundamental aspects of our living and dying. As identified at the beginning of the chapter, the intention has not been to provide the reader with comprehensive details on each aspect, but rather to provide an entry, a starting point and some 'food for thought'. In order to gain a thorough and comprehensive understanding, further reading will be required alongside work-based experience in caring for someone who is dying and those important to them.

The End of Life Care Strategy declared:

> How we care for the dying is an indicator of how we care for all sick and vulnerable people. It is a measure of society as a whole and it is a litmus test for health and social care services. (Department of Health 2008a, p.10)

Good care in the dying phase requires excellent communication and assessment skills, planning, coordination of care underpinned by knowledge, compassion and sensitivity. It is a privilege, the final opportunity professionals and carers have to ensure that this unique person leaves the world peacefully and with dignity.

Further reading

Beresford, P., Adshead, L. and Croft, S. (2007) *Palliative Care, Social Work and Service Users*. London: Jessica Kingsley Publishers.

Dunphy, J. (2011) *Communication in Palliative Care: Clear Practical Advice*. Oxford: Radcliffe Publishing Ltd.

Ellershaw, J. and Wilkinson, W. (2010) *Care of the Dying: A Pathway to Excellence*. 2nd ed. Oxford: Oxford University Press.

CHAPTER 7

Care after Death

Introduction

> I had no expectations in terms of grief counselling at all...
> I felt that the professionals could tell me about the classical
> process of grief, they could tell me all about the illness, they
> could tell me all about the burial, etc... As it turned out, the
> counselling has been very useful. (Father of baby daughter,
> died aged 7 months, Lloyd [Holloway] 1997)

Good end of life care does not stop at the point of death (Department of
Health 2008a). The transition from life to death has great significance
for family, friends and carers and also for the professionals caring for
the individual. Death is inevitable and grieving a natural process but,
even when expected, the death of a close family member or friend
is likely to be emotionally distressing. If a person's wishes are not
respected, the bereaved not well supported and the impact of the death
not acknowledged, there can be long-lasting impact on how people
grieve, on their health and on their memories of the person who has
died. Professionals have an important role to play in improving the
experiences of the bereaved.

> When someone dies all staff need to follow good practice,
> which includes being responsive to family wishes. The
> support and care provided to relatives will help them cope
> with their loss. Care after death includes honouring the
> spiritual or cultural wishes of the deceased person and their
> family and carers, while ensuring legal obligations are met.
> (National End of Life Care Programme website)

Care needs to be respectful of the person who has died, affording dignity to their body and ensuring that legal and safety requirements are met. It is also important that workers be responsive to family wishes, supporting the family through the transition from life to death. The support and care provided to relatives will help them cope with their loss and reduce the risk of future physical or psychological impact. If assessment of the carers' needs has taken place, then staff will have had the opportunity to put support in place. Bereavement assessment and support prior to the death may also ease the transition from the status of relative and carer to a bereaved person with a new social status such as widow.

This chapter considers the care of the body after death to ensure that the wishes and beliefs of the deceased are respected and the information, practical and emotional support needs of bereaved family and carers are met. It reviews the current understanding of the impact of loss and models of grief and considers the legal requirements, the role of professionals, and challenges to delivering quality care. It will also look at the changing social context and draw on the literature regarding customs and practices and attempt to clarify good practice.

Care of the body

The way that the body is handled demonstrates respect for the person who has died and the attitudes and behaviour of staff can play a significant part in honouring their integrity and dignity. There are many tasks to be carried out in care after death that are delivered by a range of professionals and staff working together with the family and carers. Any wishes for donation of organs, tissues or body parts need to be honoured. These wishes may have been ascertained prior to death, for example, by the person registering and carrying a donor card. If the deceased has made it clear that they do, or do not, wish their organs or tissue to be donated, this wish must be respected. If the wishes of the donor are not known, the Human Tissue Act 2004 permits consent from the person's next of kin or nominated representative.

Some of these tasks are legal requirements and others are dependent on the wishes and preferences of the person who has died and their family and carers. We live in a multicultural society and delivering care that is sensitive to the cultural and religious needs of the dying person and their family or carers is an essential part of care after death (National End of Life Care Programme 2009a). Safety issues also need to be taken into consideration to protect those who come into contact with the body. It is the doctor in charge of the person's care who is responsible for identifying and communicating any potential hazards. These include notifiable infections and implantable devices.

Legal requirements

Most countries have legal requirements following a death. In England confirmation or verification of the death is required. The Academy of Medical Royal Colleges' code of practice (AoMRC 2008) states that the death should be verified as soon as possible by a doctor or qualified nurse. Determination of the medical cause of death is also required and a Medical Certificate of the Cause of Death (MCCD) has to be completed before the body can be transferred to a funeral director or the death registered. A doctor who provided care during the last illness will usually certify the cause of death. Once the cause of death has been determined, the death must be registered with the Registrar of Births Marriages and Deaths, usually within five days of the death, and a death certificate issued. This is a permanent legal record of the death.

There are circumstances where the death needs to be referred to the coroner in order to confirm or determine the cause of death (Ministry of Justice 2012). Currently in England, around 46 per cent of all deaths are referred to the coroner. The coroner is a senior and independent judicial officer who determines whether a post-mortem examination or inquests are required. If the coroner decides that the medical cause of death is not clear, then a post-mortem examination will be carried out by a pathologist. A post-mortem, also known as an autopsy, is the examination of a body to determine the cause of death. If the cause of death remains unknown after the post-mortem, if there is cause for the coroner to suspect that the deceased died a violent or unnatural death or if the death occurred in custody, the coroner will order an inquest. An inquest is a formal court hearing to examine the circumstances of the death to establish who has died and the circumstances, time and place of the death. Such procedures can be traumatic for the family and a recent Australian study questioned the need for deaths at home to be treated as 'sudden' and 'unexplained' when the person in question had been suffering from a life-limiting condition in which death could reasonably be expected (Hughes 2013).

☞   STOP AND THINK!

What impact might a post-mortem have for the family? What can I do to make this easier?

Box 7.1 Deaths requiring coronial investigation

- No doctor attended the deceased during his or her last illness.

- Although a doctor attended during the last illness the deceased was not seen either within the last 14 days before death nor after death.

- The cause of death appears unknown.

- The death occurred during an operation or before recovery from the effects of an anaesthetic.

- The death occurred at work or was due to industrial disease or poisoning.

- The death was sudden or unexpected.

- The death was unnatural.

- The death was due to violence or neglect.

- The death was in other suspicious circumstances.

- The death occurred in prison, police custody or other state detention.

Source: 'A guide to coroners and inquests and charter for coroner services', Ministry of Justice (2012)

As part of the response to the recommendations of the Shipman Inquiry (Home Secretary 2007) the UK Ministry of Justice is currently reforming the coronial service. The proposed changes will require the certified cause of all deaths that are not investigated by a coroner to be independently scrutinised and confirmed by a locally appointed medical examiner. New legislation to support the changes is expected in 2014.

Preparation of the body

The physical procedures to prepare a body for burial or cremation are now termed 'personal care after death'. National guidance has been developed in England to support staff in this role (National End of Life Care Programme 2011c). In hospitals this task is usually carried out by registered nurses but in others settings such as care homes, hospices and people's own homes, it may be carried out by carers, social care staff, GPs/family doctors or funeral directors. The responsibility for this role has changed over time. At the beginning of the twentieth century it was a key task of the family and community members, often in connection with the religious community. As death became more medicalised, the role moved to the nurse in hospitals or hospices. This has resulted in distancing the bereaved from death rituals, including the physical preparation of the body, and only after the body has been 'cleaned, plugged and wrapped' by professionals can it be restored to the family (Hockey *et al.* 2010).

Some families and carers may want to participate in caring for the body and should have the opportunity and be supported to do so if they wish. There may be spiritual, religious, cultural or practical choices or requirements the dying person and their family or carers may have for the time of death or afterwards. Specific wishes may have been included in the advance care planning (ACP) process or made nearer to the point of death. Staff can help these to be achieved by encouraging communication and discussions and keeping a flexible approach. This is particularly important in cases where the person's body needs to be released urgently for burial or cremation. The overarching principle is to ensure the privacy and dignity of the deceased person.

Box 7.2 Religious rituals in Judaism

Upon the death, the eyes are closed, the body is covered and candles may be lit next to it. The candle is symbolic of the human soul and of God's eternal presence. Some choose to place the body on the floor. From the moment of death, there is a tradition of accompanying the body so that the deceased is not left alone. Many Jewish communities have a special group of volunteers responsible for washing the body and preparing it for burial in accordance with Jewish custom. There are three distinct parts: cleansing, purification with a cascade of water to wash away all the suffering of the last periods of their lives and dressing the body in white shrouds. Everybody, rich or poor, young or old, religious or nonreligious, is buried in the same garments. The body is then placed in a coffin and burial or cremation takes place as soon as possible after death. Just before the funeral, close relatives of the deceased observe the rite of k'riah – the tearing of a garment as a symbol of grief.

Transitions and rituals

When a loved one dies, the bereaved has to manage the transition from life to death and the change of their relationship with the deceased. Use of rituals after death to facilitate this transition (status passage) was described by Van Gennep (1909, 1960). He described three stages for passing from one status to the other: separation from the first status, followed by a liminal phase before integration into the new status. Each stage is marked by rites and rituals that facilitate the transition. The concept of liminality is used to explain the period of time following death during which certain rituals were performed and after which the deceased could be regarded as 'finally dead' (Holloway 2007). This 'passage' or state of liminality also allows people to assume new identities such as 'widow' (Hockey et al. 2010).

Box 7.3 The transition from life to death

When my mother died, although we'd all been anticipating it for several months, it still came as a huge shock. This was because we had reached a stage of living one day at a time and kept hoping for another day – probably because it was just too painful to consider an alternative. In that way we had adjusted to our 'very ill' mother and sharing time and thoughts with her although she couldn't communicate. We didn't really accept that death was so imminent. This meant that when she drew her last breath, there was a sudden realisation that it was an ending. It felt a huge step and was so final.

Source: Susan, daughter

Metaphors such as sleep and journeying are frequently used to describe the liminal state. Gell (1998) describes how the deceased's personal belongings, such as clothing or jewellery, can become extensions or representations of the person. Photographs can play an important role in grief as they facilitate continuing bonds with the person who has died and can be a trigger for talking about them with others. Death and the corpse remind people of their own mortality and the uncertainty of timing of death. It may also bring back memories of the deaths of others that were close to them. Rituals associated with death and mourning are an important way to help restore order and orderly progression between states (Hockey *et al.* 2010; Kanitsaki 2002). They include viewing the body, funerals, tending the grave, retention of ashes and memorials. The rituals people use will depend on the practices, customs and traditions that reflect their specific philosophies, religion, beliefs and values. Holloway (2007) identifies the secularisation of western society in the twentieth century as a major factor that has undermined the reliance on traditional religious practices surrounding death and dying with a consequent loss of ritual to support the dying, the bereaved and the community.

Funerals and memorials

Funerals and memorials represent a way to pay our respects to, say goodbye to and celebrate the life of the person who has died. They give people an opportunity to grieve both individually and collectively, allowing people to express grief and draw strength from other people who knew the deceased.

The Co-operative Funeralcare survey 2011 reports that funerals across the UK are undergoing a fundamental change. The majority of English funerals still follow a traditional religious format but there is a shift towards contemporary, more personalised services and an increasing number of humanist funerals. The style in general is becoming less sombre with the focus on celebration of the life rather than mourning and families are increasingly adding personal touches to arrange unique and uplifting funerals for their loved ones.

As well as the more traditional models for remembering the dead, such as newspaper obituaries and condolence books, other contemporary rituals are emerging including roadside memorials, memorial websites and internet obituaries (virtual cemeteries). New trends include the use of cremated ashes for tattooing the body with a permanent reminder and the setting up of temporary memorial sites (Linda Woodhead 2013). These modern practices reflect the ongoing relationship with the dead.

Grief and mourning

Grief is a universal response to the death and loss of a loved one. It is an individual experience resulting from the physical loss of the person and there is no 'normal' pattern although there may be common responses. Mourning refers to the behaviours people engage in (including those accompanied by traditional rituals as discussed above) and these may be 'socially defined and publicly recognised' (Holloway 2007, p.66). Although grief is predominantly an emotional and psychological response, it can also affect physical health, behaviour and thinking. Grief is influenced by many factors including circumstances of the death, the relationship with the deceased, personality, age, cultural background, religious beliefs, previous experiences and coping strategies (see Box 7.4). Grief is also shaped by the social context with the interpersonal support received and sociocultural factors including rituals, practices and attitudes towards death and bereavement, all impacting on the experience.

Immediately following a death, people may feel emotions such as shock, numbness, guilt, anger, fear or confusion. There may also be physical reactions such as insomnia and loss of appetite. Bereavement can trigger memories and pain from previous losses and, for some, their personal faith and beliefs may be challenged.

☞   STOP AND THINK!

Is there anything I can do as a professional to help prepare a family for the shock of the death?

Depending on the circumstances of the death, the bereaved may have experienced anticipatory grief – a reaction that occurs in anticipation of an impending loss. There may be many points in the disease trajectory when family and carers experience anticipatory grief and staff may have the opportunity to open discussions with the family and also to facilitate conversations between the individual and their family. The better prepared the family are for the death, with unfinished business resolved, the smaller the risk of a poor bereavement outcome (Barry *et al.* 2002).

Theoretical models of grief

Over the years many theoretical models of grief have been described. The traditional psychological model constructs grief as a 'severing of ties' which is approached as a process of 'letting go and moving on' (Valentine 2006). Grief has also been considered a condition that needs treating and the notion of recovery and resolution could be considered to medicalise grief; Engel (1961) likened grief to a disease. Stage or process models have also been described (Bowlby 1980; Parkes 1975, Worden 1991). These models organise grief-related symptoms into phases or stages, suggesting that grief is a process that leads to recovery. Other models offer a more flexible approach. The Dual Process model (Stroebe and Schut 1999) outlines two concurrent activities required for 'recovery' – loss and restoration – and Machin's

Range of Response to Loss model (Relf *et al.* 2010) considers the balance between emotions and more cognitive coping factors.

More recently, there has been greater recognition of the impact of diversity within cultures and between individuals (Valentine 2006) and models that consider the continuing relationship with those that have died. Walter (1996) describes a model of grief whereby the bereaved construct a personal biography that places and keeps the dead within their lives. The theory of 'continuing bonds', which marks a shift from the once-popular 'stage theories' of grief, describes the relationships that people maintain with their dead (Klass *et al.* 1996) and also takes greater account of social and cultural context. The modern shift of perception finds that grief is not necessarily time limited, with the dead continuing to influence the lives of the living and so dismantling the boundaries between life and death (Valentine 2006). In fact, the research evidence over the last two decades recognises grief as a complex, multidimensional phenomenon influenced by a variety of external factors. Social, cultural and religious worldviews all influence grief reactions, informing the individual response to death (Sheehy 2013).

Recognition of the complexity of grief and the influence of multiple external factors has important implications for professionals who work in end of life care. An awareness and understanding of the grief process and the factors that influence bereavement together with an open approach will help staff to support the range of needs of the bereaved.

Complicated grief

Although grief is painful, most people manage to adapt to this life transition, but for some additional support is required. Stage and process models view grief as a pathway that moves the bereaved on, leaving the deceased behind, and allows them to form new attachments. In this way the concept of 'normal grief' and 'complicated grief' has developed where the continuation of grief becomes 'abnormal' and medicalised as a complicated grief disorder. Complicated grief has been described as a state in which the bereaved person is significantly and functionally impaired by prolonged grief symptoms for a period longer than is expected (Shear 2011). An individual's culture plays a large role in determining what is a complicated or inappropriate pattern of grief, and it is necessary to consider cultural norms before reaching a diagnosis. Despite the considerable research on the subject, some argue that complicated grief remains poorly defined without formal diagnosis (Arthur *et al.* 2011). However, there is general agreement that some people are at higher risk of experiencing complicated grief, which can impact on their mental and physical health. Knowing when to intervene and offer professional help to a bereaved carer can be difficult. Factors that increase a person's vulnerability have been identified which, together with assessment of individual resilience and coping styles, may guide professionals in assessing those who might benefit from professional help.

People who suffer complicated grief may find it more difficult to adjust to life without the person who has died and they may be at increased risk of persistent physical and mental health problems (Stroebe *et al.* 2001) with evidence of increased mortality from heart disease and increased prevalence of psychiatric illness (Arthur *et al.* 2011; Parkes 1998).

Box 7.4 Factors that increase vulnerability

1. The circumstances of the death. The death of someone close to us is distressing. Stress and vulnerability increase if carers experience aspects of the patient's care as problematic, or if the illness and death are particularly disturbing – for example, unexpected deaths, traumatic loss, late prognosis and lack of compassion.

2. Personal vulnerability. The meaning of the lost relationship has a key influence on the experience of grief. The more the carer is dependent on the patient for their well-being, the greater the potential disruption. Conversely, carers who have had a highly ambivalent relationship with the deceased may also experience high levels of distress including high levels of guilt. Carers with

poor physical health or a history of anxiety, depression or other mental health problems may also be more vulnerable.

3. Availability of social support. People who are socially isolated or who perceive support as unhelpful may experience more difficulties in bereavement. Family tensions may cause further distress. Some people's grief may be less socially validated, e.g. following suicide, illnesses such as HIV or where the relationship is stigmatised or unrecognised such as homosexual partners and secret relationships.

4. Anticipatory grieving. Patients and carers experience grief as they grapple with the impact of a life-limiting illness. This is normal and may help people prepare for impending loss. Carers who are looking after someone with an advancing disease may anticipate the losses they have yet to experience and think about how they will cope. The ability to anticipate and to plan for the future can be helpful but for some people this way of coping is anathema; it can be seen as destroying hope and as hastening the loss.

5. Concurrent events. Some people may be experiencing multiple losses, perhaps due to a road accident or if there have been significant losses in the past. Similarly, concurrent life events such as a lack of economic resources, redundancy or the breakdown of a marriage or long-term relationship increase stress and strain coping resources.

Source: compiled from Machin 2007; Relf 2008; Relf *et al.* 2010; Stroebe *et al.* 2006.

Supporting the bereaved

Each person will experience grief in their own way and this makes assessment of their bereavement needs complex. Holistic assessment of the bereaved, including practical, emotional, information, spiritual and physical needs, is a continuous process that may commence prior to death of the person. Support prior to the death will help carers to prepare for the impending loss of the person and may help to eradicate any unnecessary fears and uncertainty. Support plans for the bereaved that can be implemented without delay are useful for professionals at the time of the death.

There are a range of formal risk assessment tools that aim to identify those at increased risk of or experiencing a complicated or prolonged grief reaction. It has been difficult to formulate robust, evidence-based tools and the ability of these tools to predict those who will benefit from bereavement intervention is unproven. A review of assessment tools (Agnew *et al.* 2010) found they lacked specificity and recommended that they should not be used as stand-alone tools. They can, however, be useful for experienced staff when integrated with recognition of day-to-day coping and support needs. An understanding of the various models of grief and identification of people's natural coping strategies will also support staff to recognise those at risk of complicated grief.

☛   STOP AND THINK!

When I assess the family's bereavement needs, what do I take into account?

Bereavement support is an essential component of good end of life care. Each loss is unique and sensitive and compassionate care tailored to the bereaved person is important. The first 48 hours following the death of someone close can be one of the most bewildering and emotive times in a person's life with legal requirements for certification and registration competing with emotional responses to loss (Chaplin 2012). Many people will not have experienced a death before and will not understand the legal and practical requirements nor may they be prepared for the emotional impact.

The right support at the right time
If supported well at this time, the vast majority of people will not require formal grief counselling. Providing the bereaved with information

and guidance on the practical procedures, what to expect and when and how to access more support will enable them to access the level of support that they need. It will also facilitate early identification of those who may need professional support.

The bereaved may have a variety of needs which include information and guidance and practical, financial, social, emotional and spiritual support. These needs may be immediate or emerge over time. Social networks provide the main source of support for most people who feel they do not need formal bereavement services (Arthur *et al.* 2011 and Wimpenny 2006). Acknowledgement of their loss and an understanding of bereavement and what to expect together with information about access to additional support, if needed, is all that the majority of people need or want. Very few people request or make use of professional support. In England additional bereavement support is mainly provided by self-help groups and the voluntary sector.

Effectiveness of bereavement support

At present, there is little scientific evidence of the effectiveness of formal bereavement support and no evidence to support the universal provision of intensive bereavement interventions (Arthur *et al.* 2011). Interventions have been found to be more effective for those who self-select for help (Allumbaugh and Hoyt 2003), for people in high risk categories for bereavement-related problems and for those already suffering from clinical depression, anxiety or other bereavement-related disorders. It appears that, with the help of family and friends, most people are able to work through and integrate their loss without any formal intervention. Where more support is required, the optimal timing may be between 6 and 18 months after a death (Jordon and Neimeyer 2003) but this still needs to be empirically evaluated. We should, however, bear in mind that for some people, the experience of grief may reduce the likelihood of them recognising their need and seeking help (Arthur *et al.* 2011). The evidence to date supports the three component model of bereavement support (NICE 2004). (See Box 7.5)

Box 7.5 The three-component model of bereavement (NICE 2004)

Component 1: Grief is a normal reaction to bereavement and most people manage without professional intervention by drawing on their own coping mechanisms and the support from family, friends and community networks in their lives. All bereaved people should be offered information about the experience of bereavement and how to access other forms of support.

Component 2: Some people who are bereaved may require more support over and above that which family and friends can provide and a more formal opportunity to review and reflect on their experience of loss. This support may include but is not limited to community health and social care services, voluntary groups, self-help groups and spiritual and faith groups and may or may not include some professional support. Clear referral processes to Component 3 interventions must be in place when cases involve more complex needs emerge.

Component 3: A smaller number of people may find it more difficult to adjust to their loss and experience complex grief with persisting physical and mental health problems and need therapeutic interventions. Early recognition and referral is essential.

Note: This guidance was developed for adults with cancer but the model can be applied to all adults who are bereaved, regardless of the cause.

Support services

Building relationships with the family and carers, open communication and good support during the dying phase will have a positive effect on the subsequent experience of bereavement. People are likely to feel shock and sometimes anger, guilt and numbness immediately following a death and this is a time when they need support. It is often considered that some people are better than others at supporting the bereaved but training and education can give staff the required confidence and skills (National End of Life Care Programme 2009b). Sensitive communication that demonstrates compassion and empathy and that maintains dignity and respect for both the person that has died and for the family is important and is essential to accept the death and look back on the experience with positive feelings. Showing the smallest acts of kindness – for example, personally addressed condolence cards, using discreet property bags to return the deceased's personal belongings and holding regular remembrance services – can make an enormous difference.

Wider family members and carers may want to be partners in care after death but may not know how and may feel intimidated. An inclusive approach where staff are sensitive and responsive to the family members' needs will help the family to be involved as little or as much as they wish. Getting the balance right between being readily available if required but giving the family their privacy will also help to empower the family. It is helpful to understand the variation in grief and coping reactions, with emotional outbursts being as normal as withdrawal, silence and numbness.

Satisfaction with the care that has been provided throughout and especially in the last few days and at time of death will impact on the family's experience of care after death. A wide range of professionals are often involved in caring for the person and the family and coordination and collaboration of services makes a difference. Studies show that continuity of care into bereavement is perceived by relatives as important (Lord and Pockett 1998). Deaths that involve inquests or investigations can be especially stressful for family and carers. Setting up a fast-track system to a bereavement support agency offering longer-term support by specialist bereavement support workers in the community has been found to be beneficial (Chaplin 2012).

Provision of information

Many people will not have experienced a death before or understand the legal and practical requirements. This can feel bewildering and overwhelming at a time when people are very vulnerable. Information given to the bereaved immediately at time of death and shortly afterwards is helpful (National End of Life Care Programme 2011a). Clear understanding of what happens next, the legal and statutory requirements, signposting to funeral services and financial and practical support will help the bereaved to make plans.

In addition, information on the emotional impact of loss, grief and possible physical reactions such as insomnia and appetite loss will prepare people in advance and so reduce anxiety should they experience these reactions. Signposting to national and local bereavement support services together with information about risk factors will facilitate prompt access to additional bereavement support if required. There is much information to be conveyed and as people are likely to be emotionally fragile, the provision of written information for families to take away with them in a range of formats to meet varying population needs is helpful. Written information should be used to consolidate, not replace, verbal communication (National End of Life Care Programme 2011). This can be done through provision of a dedicated website and helpline to improve access to information and guidance and to support relatives and friends with any questions about practical concerns such as funeral arrangements, financial concerns and legal questions.

Most families and carers in England use a funeral director to make arrangements for the funeral. The funeral director will discuss family wishes for care of the body, the funeral or cremation and help with decisions on the ashes and on memorials. Planning the funeral may start before death as families come to terms with an imminent death. Sometimes, the dying person may want to be involved to ease the burden on family or to ensure that their personal views are reflected but often planning does not start until after the death. Decisions and arrangements often have to be completed in a very tight timescale at a time when family and carers may be in shock and feeling overwhelmed emotionally. Some people find that the focus on these practical tasks helps them to cope with the immediate post-death period (see Box 7.6).

Box 7.6 An integrated support programme

A funeral director, a local hospice and the community bereavement support group work together to provide practical and emotional support to the bereaved. Weekly sessions include 'Cooking for one', 'Looking after yourself', 'A guide to finances' and 'The bereavement journey – am I normal?' These sessions also provide a supportive forum for recently bereaved people to discuss their experiences.

Emotional support

People draw primarily on support from their family, friends and social networks if available but staff also play an important role in providing emotional support immediately following death. It is known that the bereaved find comfort in acknowledgement of the death and recognition of their grief (Arthur *et al.* 2011). Emotional needs vary from person to person and people who have compassion, are adaptable, have good listening skills and who use sensitive and supportive communication will best support the bereaved. Unfortunately, some people find it difficult to interact with the bereaved and avoid these conversations. A study by Bath (2009) found that people's previous experience and beliefs about their effectiveness and competence to support a person were the most important predictors of their willingness to offer support.

Bereavement support services are often provided by volunteers, social, religious, cultural or community groups (see, for example, Box 7.7). These may be group peer-support sessions or one-to-one support. In most cases these services will be supervised by trained professionals. Availability of a range of services will provide for varying needs between individuals and over time. Complicated and prolonged grief is likely to need professional input (Arthur *et al.* 2011). Therapeutic services are delivered by specialist staff and may be delivered as one-to-one therapy, group therapy and couple or family therapy. Knowledge of the available services and the referral processes will help the bereaved access the appropriate support. Boxese 7.6 and 7.7 are good practice examples for supporting the bereaved.

Box 7.7 Telephone follow-up calls

Bereavement staff telephone bereaved relatives four weeks after the death to check how they are coping and to ask whether they have any questions or concerns. The majority require only one follow-up call as people state they are OK and being supported by friends and family but a small minority require additional help. It is believed that these follow-up calls facilitate early intervention and can resolve situations that, if not addressed, could have a lasting impact for the bereaved.

☞   STOP AND THINK

Reflect on your experiences of communication with people recently bereaved. What went well? What could have been better?

Spiritual support

There is evidence that indicates that spirituality, including religion, is an important coping mechanism for many approaching the end of life (Holloway *et al.* 2011) and also for those close to them. Holistic care incorporates spiritual well-being and sees this as a responsibility of all those providing care.

Spirituality can be described as the way in which people understand and live their lives in relation to their core beliefs and values and their perception of meaning of life and death (Marie Curie 2003). Meaning-making is a core concept in understandings of contemporary spirituality and also in current grief and bereavement theory (Holloway et al. 2013). A death may result in a major life change and loss for the bereaved. There may also be other less visible or acknowledged losses such as income, career, status, identity, freedom and lifestyle, as well as unfulfilled expectations or dreams. Death and bereavement can challenge people's values and beliefs and spiritual support may be helpful.

Spiritual support needs to be tailored to individual needs, beliefs and values. In some circumstances the support may have a religious focus or component but not for all. Spiritual support may include recognition of the impact of bereavement on a person's beliefs and values, listening, talking, story-construction and counselling. In England, the chaplaincy has had a key role in spiritual support of the dying and bereaved. Over recent years, their role has changed in line with the movement towards secularisation and chaplains generally support those of all faiths and those without faith (Holloway et al. 2011). The nursing profession also has a long association with spirituality with many hospices associated with religious orders. Spiritual care models have been developed (Holloway et al. 2011) aiming to support all staff to incorporate spiritual support into the everyday context of care.

Challenges

There are a number of issues that may make provision of care after death particularly challenging.

Conflict

A major goal for quality care after death is to meet the needs and preferences of both the deceased person and their family members. However, family conflict may be present in many deaths (Kramer and Yonker 2011). Staff may find themselves torn between responding to the wishes and needs of the bereaved and at the same time taking into account the deceased person's wishes for their care after death. Clarity over people's wishes made before death reduces the risk of family disagreements and conflict but emotional distress, anxiety and other pressures can contribute to misunderstandings and conflict between staff and the family and between family members. This increases distress for the family and professionals. Holding family meetings may help to build trust, promote reciprocal understanding of needs and preferences and enhance communication between family, patient and staff (Kramer and Yonker 2011). It is important in bereavement support to remember that conflict between family members can develop over time as different ways of grieving emerge and members find it more difficult to find support from each other (Breen and O'Connor 2011).

Meeting cultural/religious and spiritual needs

In a multicultural society and in modern times, one size definitely does not fit all. Efforts to understand variations in experiences of grief in different cultures found that practitioners with a western 'worldview' often consider other beliefs, practices and values as irrational or inferior (Valentine 2006). The general approach to addressing this has been by providing professionals with information about cultural practices. However, this goes only partway in achieving the change in approach required to achieve culturally sensitive and competent practice which fully embraces diversity (Holloway 2006). Building respectful relationships and fully involving the person and family in identifying and communicating their needs will help to support meaningful family and community connections, and ultimately reinforce cultural meaning, affirm self-identity and integrity and instil a sense of belonging.

Vulnerable groups

There are some groups that may find it more difficult to access the support they need. Older bereaved people may experience barriers to accessing adequate support. In part, this can be because with increasing age, death becomes so much a cultural norm and the impact is not always recognised. Also, older people may feel less able to cope with the life-changing impact of the death of a loved one or friend and the death may come at a time when previously reliable support systems have become weakened or disappeared. Older people may have been dependent on the person who has died for support, company and social identity and there may be financial implications that add to their stress (Cruse Bereavement Care undated).

There are particular challenges to communicating with and supporting those with dementia and learning disabilities to be as fully involved as they wish. Family members may be anxious about the impact and wish to 'protect' them from knowledge of the death. This can result in exclusion and may impact adversely on their grief. Access to additional bereavement support and specialist bereavement support may be required.

Effects of death on staff

We should not forget that a death can also be difficult for staff, especially for those who have had closer and longer relationships with the person (Rickerson 2005). A literature review exploring the impact of deaths in a hospital setting found nurses were affected both in their work environment and outside of work (Wilson and Kirschbaum 2011).

For non-palliative care medical staff, a patient's death following a long illness may be experienced as a personal and professional failure with feelings of frustration and powerlessness. If not acknowledged and addressed these emotions may result in distress, disengagement, burnout, and poor judgment (Diane *et al.* 2001). Education and training programmes around grief theory and peer support have been found to be helpful for developing coping strategies (Arthur *et al.* 2011).

Death as taboo

In the early 1900s, nearly all deaths occurred in the home. Death was familiar and very much a part of our everyday lives. Caring for the sick and dying was the responsibility of family, friends and neighbours, as were the laying out of the dead and preparations for the funeral. The medicalisation of death led to changes in usual place of death, with declining numbers of people dying in their own home and the majority of deaths occurrng in hospital.

The End of Life Care Strategy (Department of Health 2008a) highlighted the taboo in England about discussing death and dying. This aligns with Geoffrey Gorer's work; Gorer introduced the idea of the *stigma* of grief (Gorer 1965), which impacts on the way that staff and the community are able to support the bereaved. This taboo means that too many people have not discussed or shared their wishes on how they wish to be cared for at the end of life. In addition, people may find it difficult to talk to those that have been bereaved and may avoid them altogether, leaving them to grieve in isolation. The avoidance may be implicit by ignoring or failing to acknowledge the loss or changing the topic of conversation, or may be explicit by avoiding all contact with the bereaved. This lack of openness in discussion about death and dying in our society can impact on the bereavement experience and raises the risk of traumatic bereavement.

Environments of care

Deaths may be either expected or sudden and can occur in any setting. Currently, the majority of deaths occur in hospital, although this is beginning to change (Gomes *et al.* 2011). Most people state that they would prefer to die at home and few wish to die in hospital. Among those living in care settings such as care homes, prisons or hostels, many consider these to be their home. Maintaining privacy and dignity in these settings can be a challenge.

The physical environment can have a direct impact on the experience of care and the surroundings in which people see a loved one for the last time leaves a powerful memory. An environment that allows privacy and maintains the dignity of the person that has died is important (see Box 7.8). In addition, appropriate space for family and friends to sit quietly and talk to one another or to staff may make it easier for the bereaved to express their grief freely and for people to support one another. A bereavement suite away from clinical areas is ideal.

Some environments pose particular challenges to delivery of quality end of life care, providing privacy, maintaining dignity and supporting family and carers. These include busy A and E departments, hostels and prisons where it may be more difficult for staff to sensitively support the bereaved and manage practical tasks. For example, the way that a person's possessions are handled has an immediate impact and may also impact on subsequent bereavement (Waller 2008).

☞   STOP AND THINK!

How might the family feel if a person's belongings were handed over in a black plastic bag?

Box 7.8 A caring environment

A dedicated bereavement suite was built to provide a quiet and private space where relatives can collect the death certificate and personal belongings. It can be used for conversations with the doctor or nurses when required. The new suite was developed in partnership with patients and relatives and was supported by donations from the Friends of the Hospital. The suite has a contemporary design with wooden floor and large glass doors opening onto a courtyard with a small fountain. Art works have been donated by a local artist and the Cubs planted spring bulbs in the flower bed. The atmosphere is quiet, peaceful and welcoming and helps relatives to feel valued.

Conclusion

Care after death is an essential component of quality end of life care. There are many tasks to be carried out immediately following a death; these include preparation of the body for burial or cremation and complying with safety and legal requirements, in addition to providing support to the family and carers.

All those who come into contact with the bereaved have a role to play in supporting them through the transition between life and death. The support and care provided in the immediate period following a death can impact on the way that people cope with loss and can reduce the risk of future health problems. Supporting relatives can be challenging. When there have been open discussions prior to death and plans put in place, it can often be easier.

Changes in society over the last 50 years require new care approaches. England is a multicultural society that requires flexible and open attitudes to ensure that the wishes of the person that has died and their family can be met. It is helpful to recognise the role of rituals in supporting the transition from life to death and we can see evidence of a shift in practices towards contemporary, more personalised funerals and a less sombre style with the focus on celebration of the person's life.

We now have a better understanding of the complexities and the individuality of grief and recognise the importance of compassion and sensitive communication. The bereaved appreciate acknowledgement of their loss and the impact it has. Most bereaved require information and direction about the tasks that are required following a death but then draw on their personal sources of support and social networks. It is important that those who require more support are identified and appropriate care put in place.

This final step in the pathway is enormously important and can be very rewarding for the staff who provide this care and help to achieve a good death. Good care after death will be supported by the quality of end of life care provided at earlier stages of the pathway. If advance care planning has taken place, the wishes and needs of the person and their family and carers may be known. A continuum of the care pathway approach is recommended for providing good quality care after death. This is an essential component of good end of life care and cannot be seen as a separate issue. Each loss is unique and sensitive and compassionate care matched to the individual is needed. We should always remember that though our responsibilities as professionals may have come to an end, a new journey for those who have been bereaved is only just beginning.

Further reading

Arthur, A., Wilson, E., James, M., Stanton, W. and Seymour, J. (2011) 'Bereavement care services: a synthesis of the literature.' Department of Health. Available at www.gov.uk/government/uploads/system/uploads/attachment_data/file/147509/Department of Health_123810.pdf, accessed on 21 May 2013.

Dying Matters. 'Handling bereavement.' Available at www.dyingmatters.org/page/handling-bereavement, accessed 21 May 2013.

Relf, M., Machin, L. and Archer, N. (2010) Guidance for Bereavement Needs Assessment in Palliative Care, 2nd edition. London: Help the Hospices. Available at www.helpthehospices.org.uk, accessed 9 August 2013.

CHAPTER 8

Quality End of Life Care for All

Introduction

Over the last decade we have seen a dramatic expansion of palliative care from its early focus on end-stage cancer to a significantly broader focus on end of life care for all. We now understand that the 'good death' means 'dying well' and this implies a process of *living* through the end stage of life; and since every individual's life is so different, so a good death for one person may reflect different values and priorities than for another. However, the case studies used throughout this book also tell a common story. People want to be listened to and treated with dignity and respect; they, and the professionals around them, find it difficult to talk about dying but experience it as an empowering process when they do; people who are approaching the end of life, with their families, want to be in control of decisions about their care but they need good information and professional expertise to make and support those decisions and to realise their choices; they do not have time or energy to spend on trying to make services join up or repeatedly explaining what their problems are; they need to feel confident that wherever and whenever they need care it will be of the highest possible standard; above all, they need to feel that their life, their death and their loss is important to the people caring for them, that they are treated with compassion and valued.

These common components of 'dying well' apply to everyone approaching the end of life, irrespective of age, gender, health condition or disability, sexual orientation, culture or socio-economic status. They are reflected in the six steps of the end of life care pathway which the preceding chapters have explored. The pathway is a guide, an aide-mémoire, for practitioners, service managers and policy makers to enable us to develop, monitor and improve the end of life care that we are delivering. However, what should always be remembered is that each person's pathway is their own, shaped by their own unique set of characteristics and circumstances. If someone is not ready to discuss their wishes until they are well on the way with their care pathway, for example, we should take time at that point to revisit plans and listen to the wishes and worries, hopes and fears of the person whose end of life journey this is.

There are some excellent examples of end of life care services and innovations contained within each chapter of this book that, intuitively, suggest that the focus on end of life care that we have seen in England since the launch of the national Strategy in 2008 is making a difference to the quality of people's last months, weeks and days of life. However, certain core indicators are systematically reviewed annually. These are features of end of life that bear international comparison since they are commonly recognised to reflect quality end of life care (Institute of Medicine 2003; Economist Intelligence Unit 2010). This chapter will briefly review the progress made against these indicators before concluding by exploring some of the issues and themes that look set to shape the future of end of life care.

Place of death

The one measure that is constantly highlighted is the relationship between preferred place of care and the actual place of death. Just prior to the launch of the End of Life Care Strategy, the National Audit Commission had reported that whilst the majority of people say that they should prefer to die at home, in fact 58 per cent died in hospital and only 19 per cent at home (NAO 2008). Meanwhile, reporting that annual deaths were expected to rise by 17 per cent between 2012 and 2030, Gomes and Higginson predicted that on the basis of analysing trends in place of death, fewer than 10 per cent of those deaths would be at home if present trends continued (Gomes and Higginson 2009).

We now take a more nuanced look at this issue. First, instead of collecting statistics on deaths at home (meaning a private residence) the significant unit of care is regarded as 'usual place of residence', reflecting the fact that for the immediate and possibly medium-term future, many people will have been in a long-term residential care facility for a number of years and this has become their home. Thus, another set of statistics is equally important; this charts the numbers who die in care homes and other supported living facilities rather than being moved into hospital because of some acute care episode that ends in their death. Figures produced by the National End of Life Care Intelligence Network (NEoLCIN 2012) show that in 2010, 53 per cent of people died in hospital, 21 per cent in their own home (private residence) and 18 per cent in care homes, indicating a steady upward trend of death in usual place of residence (DIUPR).

Data concerning preferences of place of care and place of death is collected through the Electronic Palliative Care Coordination System (EPaCCS – see Chapter 4) and of those who have such a record, 47 per cent expressed a preference to die at home, 33 per cent in a hospice, 29 per cent in a care home and 1 per cent in hospital. This compares with a telephone survey of the general population aged 16 years and over, in which home emerged as the most preferred place of death (63%) with hospice the second preference (29%); however, for those aged 75 and over, preference for home had decreased to 45 per cent and preference for hospice had increased. A significant figure when considering the impact of end of life care tools is that 76 per cent of people who had died with an EPaCCS record in place died in their preferred place, but 21 per cent did not and 8 per cent died in hospital. Further, the gap between preferred and actual place of death is highest for older people, who are the most likely to die in hospital although this figure decreases slightly to 48 per cent dying in hospital in the 90+ age group. The other group most likely to die in hospital is those from the most deprived quintile in the socio-economic index, although there will be some overlap between this and older people. Recent evidence specific to cancer patients confirms that most prefer to die at home or in a hospice, but most (48%) continue to die in hospital. However, there has been a steady downward trend in hospital deaths and an increase in home deaths (Gao *et al.* 2013).

Two points should be emphasised here. First, the trend towards death in usual place of residence combined with an encouraging degree of matching of preference to actual place of death when the person is on an integrated care plan using a coordinated electronic recording system suggests that end of life care strategies and plans are in place and having an effect at the local level. Second, too many people continue to die in hospital despite their expressed preferred place of care being home or hospice, but there are implications that hospital care continues to have a part to play in end of life care and is sometimes the preferred option. We shall explore this later in the chapter.

Care planning

Building on early evidence that end of life care planning improves the quality of life for both the person at the end of life and the carer (Wright *et al.* 2008), a major thrust of the National End of Life Care Programme's work has been to improve the instances, timing and quality of end of life care planning (see Chapter 3; also National End of Life Care Programme 2009a and 2012c). Advance care planning in particular has been demonstrated to have an impact on the quality of the care provided further down the care pathway and to reduce stress and depression in bereaved relatives (Detering *et al.* 2010). One of the reasons for this is that it enables people to express their preference for place of death and benefits carers through giving them a mandate to take decisions on the person's behalf where necessary. Advance care plans also facilitate important people being around the person in the final stage (IHM 2011).

Disease trajectories and care pathways

A lot more is now known about particular disease groups and their care pathways (NEoLCIN 2012). This enables a targeting of improvements which was not possible before this data was collected. For example, people dying of liver disease, a growing problem in the UK, predominantly (73%) die in hospital as do 65 per cent of those with respiratory disease. Perhaps surprisingly, only 25 per cent of those with dementia die in hospital (although we know that identifying dementia as underlying cause of death is problematic) (National End of Life Care Intelligence Network 2010). One particular group whose palliative care needs are largely unmet is homeless people with advanced liver disease; in fact, homeless people are an extremely vulnerable group whose unmet needs prompted the production of a Route to Success (National End of Life Care Programme 2010d).

Quality of care

Developing tools and methods to obtain detailed information about the quality of end of life care is another priority. The drive to report, measure and evaluate the overall quality of care alongside evidence on the effectiveness of clinical treatments is a significant move to achieve the vision of holistic, person-centred end of life care. Obtaining patient and service user views on the quality of end of life care received has become a regular feature of service review. The VOICES survey has been referred to in a number of places throughout this book and it has provided information on the rating of quality by care settings and locality. Hospices are consistently rated as providing excellent care on all indicators; hospitals and out-of-hours services are rated less favourably. Continuity of care is a significant factor contributing to overall quality but it has proved difficult to measure, and user-led/defined outcomes have been suggested as a possible tool (NEoLCIN 2012). A Real Time Survey using simple IT devices (work in progress under NEoLCIN) is currently being piloted in one region of England to enable patients and service users to give anonymous feedback at the point of the care episode or interaction. Another set of tools being rolled out are those that facilitate health and social care providers' self-rating and monitoring as an aid to achieving consistent quality and efficiently targeting areas for improvement (see Chapter 5).

The future of end of life care

It is possible to chart significant progress in end of life care in terms of government policy, health and social care practice and public awareness. Inevitably, as a result, new challenges have come to the fore.

Support for carers and families

Support for carers is recognised as an important aspect of end of life care, both before and after the death (see Chapter 7). However, in the drive to facilitate more people dying at home, little attention has been given to what that might mean day to day, hour by hour, for families and carers. It is too easy for healthcare professionals to assume that providing people with sophisticated equipment and access to emergency medication, with support workers and other staff popping in or leaving their mobile telephone number, covers their support needs. Rarely is it raised that for some people, particularly older partners, this burden of responsibility might be too much for them. While many people do testify to the wonderful support received from professionals and their appreciation of the fact that their loved one has been able to die at home as they had wished and they were able to enjoy a close family atmosphere to the end, other points are beginning to be raised. For example, a study in England of older people reported them saying that when home became a hospital it ceased to be home (Gott *et al.* 2004) and a recent Australian study found a number of distressing aspects of deaths in the home, including the recourse to investigatory procedures for 'unexpected' deaths (Hughes 2013). As with all aspects of end of life care, it is important to listen to carers with no preconceived agenda about the support they need or want.

Understanding well-being

Health and social care services across the developed world are becoming increasingly focused around the notion of well-being. Well-being is a much-talked about but relatively ill-defined concept. A systematic literature review of spiritual care at the end of life showed that people may experience well-being overall in their life at the same time as having a lack of well-being in some aspect (Holloway *et al.* 2011). This is an important insight for us to take into end of life care where, increasingly, we understand that living well and dying well belong together. In one sense this reiterates the hospice philosophy that people live until they die and should continue to have their wishes and choices respected to the end, but when applied to the extended phase at the end of life that is now the common experience of large groups of the population, it focuses our attention on what it means to support people living through the end phase of their life at the same time as they are dealing with a faltering body and preparing for their death. This perspective allows us to see that rehabilitation – a major focus currently in social care services in the UK – also has a role to play in end of life care services that are aimed at restoring well-being in the face of impending death. It also underlines the urgent need to reach out to marginalised communities and groups, both to increase their access to good end of life care and to open our eyes to what 'good' and 'well-being' means to them. This is the focus of the Routes to Success for LGBT people, for Prisons, and for Hostels and Homeless People. A study of sub-Saharan African communities in London (Selman *et al.* 2010) provides valuable insights into how formal services can be brought together with community resources to provide appropriate care.

Becoming mainstream

Finally, a key message from the implementation of the End of Life Care Strategy and the work of the National End of Life Care Programme in England is that end of life care is, and needs to be, moving into the mainstream. This implies continuing the efforts to raise public awareness (e.g., the Dying Matters Campaign) and developing public health approaches (Paul 2013) including the promotion of 'compassionate communities' (Brown and Walter 2013; Kellehear 2005) and an 'end of life care–friendly society' (Walker 2012). It also means embedding end of life care in mainstream service provision. In England this means, in effect, that community (primary) health services, social care services and hospitals (acute care) form a triangle of care, with good communication and effective coordination between themselves and with other service providers in the mosaic of care that makes up today's health and social care system. Hospices continue to provide excellent palliative care that is much valued by patients and families, but there is increasing recognition that hospice as a philosophy and specialist resource is too vital to be confined to a building and needs to reach out to people at the end of life in their own homes through partnerships with mainstream community health and social care services.

Hospitals also have a part to play, but should be used for planned episodes of care where their resources and expertise are best suited to the particular need, rather than for unnecessary emergency admissions (including where the need is for palliative care) which too often result in the person dying in hospital. In England, people in the last year of life currently average 2.1 hospital admissions over the year (NEoLCIN 2012) and too few are enabled to return to their usual place of residence after a serious episode such as a stroke (CVA). This compares with data from other countries indicating that the majority of older people have multiple care changes in the last year of life (Chan *et al.* 2003; Klinkenberg *et al.* 2005).

From a position where end of life care was seen to be the responsibility of health services, social care initiatives in end of life care in England are now gaining momentum, with the Association of Directors of Adult Social Services (ADASS) giving full backing to the National End of Life Care Programme's Social Care Framework (National End of Life Care Programme 2010c) and subsequent implementation initiatives. In this respect, England has trailed behind countries such as the US and Australia, where social work has been actively engaged in leading palliative and end of life care developments, but the nature of the organisation of social care support in the UK places it now in a key position. Around 30 per cent of people use some form of local government-funded social care in the last year of life and there is tentative evidence that higher social care costs at the end of life are linked to lower hospital inpatient costs (Bardsley *et al.* 2011). Importantly, those older people suffering from one or more of the diseases of old age that are the main causes of death in this age group (such as cardiovascular and respiratory problems) tend to make relatively high use of social care services, as do those with dementia and chronic mental health problems (NEoLCIN 2012). We must continue efforts to raise awareness and maintain an openness about dying and end of life care in the wider society, but we cannot expect from the general public a response that we as professionals have failed to grasp ourselves. It is imperative that quality end of life care be provided as part of routine care, as and when the individual reaches that stage in their care journey.

Conclusion

It is a testament to the success of the National End of Life Care Programme that end of life care is now addressed across all domains of health and social care services in the UK. The message that quality of life and quality in death belong together is an important one.

When life expectancy was short by comparison with today's, 'death in the midst of life' was accepted, but many people experienced neither good health in life nor a good death. The sociologists of death and dying were right to point to the personal misery and social dysfunction caused by the denial of death in society as the ultimate taboo subject and the impersonal nature of health care when medical technologies take over. For too many people in the twentieth century, dying and bereavement were lonely and painful processes.

But we have learned a lot and begun to do things better, not least because as professionals we have listened to the people whom we seek to serve as much as we have allowed ourselves to learn from our own experiences of death. Now, in the twenty-first century, we can say that end of life care is everybody's business and be confident that there will be broad accord. There is no room for complacency, however, as new challenges at individual, family and community levels emerge. We hope that you as readers are able to use this book as a firm foundation on which to build your practice in end of life care, one that is innovative, creative, flexible and responsive to the ever-changing environment of health and social care and the needs of those people you support through their end of life journey.

References

Abernethy, A.P., Wheeler, J.L. and Bull, J. (2011) 'Development of a Health Information Technology–based data system in community-based hospice and palliative care.' *American Journal of Preventive Medicine 40*, 5, Supplement 2 (May 2011), S217–S224.

Academy of Medical Royal Colleges (2008) *Code of Practice for the Diagnosis and Confirmation of Death.* London: Academy of Medical Royal Colleges.

Adams, R. (ed.) (2009) *Practising Social Work in a Complex World (2nd ed).* Hampshire: Palgrave Macmillan.

Addington-Hall, J. and McCarthy, M. (1995) 'Regional Study of Care for the Dying: methods and sample characteristics.' *Palliative Medicine 9*, 1, 27–35.

Agnew, A., Manktelow, R., Taylor, B. and Jones, L. (2010) 'Bereavement needs assessment in specialist palliative care: a review of the literature.' *Palliative Medicine 24*, 1, 46–59.

Allen, M. and Watts, T. (2012) 'Promoting health and wellbeing at the end of life: the contribution of care pathways.' *International Journal of Palliative Nursing 18*, 7, 348–354.

Allumbaugh, D. and Hoyt, W. (1999) 'Effectiveness of grief therapy: a meta-analysis.' *Journal of Counseling Psychology 46*, 3, 370–380.

Altilio, T. and Otis-Green, S. (eds) (2011) *Oxford Textbook of Palliative Social Work.* Oxford: Oxford University Press.

Altschuler, J. in Firth, P., Luff, G. and Oliviere, D. (eds) (2005) *Loss, Change and Bereavement in Palliative Care.* Berkshire: Open University Press.

Anderson, L. (2011) 'Case report: Psychosocial support for the palliative care patient.' *Wound Essentials, 6*, 84–86.

Angus, D.C., Barnato, A.E., Linde-Zwirble, W.T., Weissfeld, L.A., Watson, R.S., Ricket, T. and Rubenfeld, G.D. (2004) 'Use of intensive care at the end of life in the United States: An epidemiologic study.' *Critical Care Medicine 32*, 3, 638–643.

Anslem, A.H., Palda, V., Guest, C.B., McLean, R.F., Vachon, M.L.S., Kelner, M. and Lam-McCulloch, J. (2005) 'Barriers to communication regarding end-of-life care: Perspectives of care providers.' *Journal of Critical Care 20*, 3, 214–223.

Aries, P. (1974) *Western Attitudes Towards Death from the Middle Ages to the Present.* Baltimore: John Hopkins University Press.

Aries, P. (1981) *The Hour of Our Death.* New York: Knopf.

Arthur, A., Wilson, E., James, M., Stanton, W. and Seymour, J. (2011) 'Bereavement care services: A synthesis of the literature.' Department of Health. Available at www.gov.uk/government/uploads/system/uploads/attachment_data/file/147509/Department of Health_123810.pdf, accessed on 21 May 2013.

Association of Palliative Care Social Workers (APCSW). Available at www.apcsw.org.uk, accessed January 2013.

Baile, F., Buckman, R., Lenzi, R., Glober, G., Beale, E.A., and Kudelka, A.P. (2000) 'SPIKES – A six-step protocol for delivering bad news: Application to the patient with cancer.' *The Oncologist 5*, 4, 302–311.

Baraclough, J., Deman, G., Osborn, H. and Willmott, P. (1996) *100 Years of Health-Related Social Work 1895–1995*. Birmingham: British Association of Social Workers.

Bardsley, G., Billings, J., Chassin, L., Dixon, J., Eastmure, E., Georghiou, T., Lewis, G., Vaithiajathan, T. and Steventon, A. (2011) *Predicting Social Care Costs: a Feasibility Study*. London: The Nuffield Trust.

Barry, L.C., Kasl, S.V. and Prigerson, H.G. (2002) 'Psychiatric disorders among bereaved persons: the role of the perceived circumstances of death and preparedness for death.' *American Journal of Geriatric Psychiatry 10*, 4, 447–457.

Bath, D. (2009) 'Predicting social support for grieving persons: a theory of planned behaviour perspective.' *Death Studies 33*, 10, 869–889.

Benz, C. and Chand, D. (2012) 'Carers.' In D. Oliver (ed.) *End of Life Care in Neurological Disease*. London: Springer.

Beresford, P., Adshead, L. and Croft, S. (2007) *Palliative Care, Social Work and Service Users: Making Life Possible*. London: Jessica Kingsley Publishers.

Beresford, P., Croft, S. and Adshead, L. (2008) '"We don't see her as a social worker": a service user case study of the importance of the social worker's relationship and humanity.' *British Journal of Social Work 38*, 7, 1388–1407.

Bodenheimer, T. (2008) 'Coordinating care – a perilous journey through the health care system.' *The New England Journal of Medicine 358*, 10, 1064–1071.

BookBrowse (2013) Available at www.bookbrowse.com/quotes/detail/index.cfm?quote_number=250, accessed 16 June 2013.

Bowlby, J. (1980) *Attachment and Loss (Volume 3): Loss, Sadness and Depression*. London: Hogarth Press.

Brazil, K., Bainbridge, D. Sussman, J., Whelan, T., O'Brien, M.A. and Pyette, N. (2008) 'Providing supportive care to cancer patients: a study on inter-organizational relationships.' *International Journal of Integrated Care 8*. Available at http://www.ncbi.nlm.nih.gov/pmc/articles/PMC2254486/, accessed 28 October 2013.

Breen, L. and O'Connor, M. (2011) 'Family and social networks after bereavement: experiences of support, change and isolation.' *Journal of Family Therapy 33*, 1, 98–120.

Brewin, T. with Sparshott, M. (1996, reprint 2005) *Relating to the Relatives: Breaking Bad News, Communication and Support*. Oxford: Radcliffe Publishing.

Brooker, C. (ed.) (2002) *Churchill Livingstone's Dictionary of Nursing*, 18th ed. Edinburgh: Churchill Livingstone.

Brown, L. and Walter, T. (2013) 'Towards a social model of end of life care.' *British Journal of Social Work*, doi: 10.1093/bjsw/bct087.

Bruce, S. (1995) *Religion in Modern Britain*. Oxford: Oxford University Press.

Buckman, R. (2000) 'Communication in palliative care: a practical guide.' *Neurological Clinics 19*, 4, 989–1004.

Buntin, M.B., Burke, M.F., Hoaglin, M.C. Blumenthal, D. (2011) 'The benefits of health information technology: a review of the recent literature shows predominantly positive results.' *Health Affairs 30*, 3, 464–471.

Bury, M. (1997) *Health and Illness in a Changing Society*. London: Routledge.

Byrne, J., McNamara, P., Seymour, J. and McClinton, P. (2009) *Palliative Care in Neurological Disease: a Team Approach*. Oxford: Radcliffe Publishing.

Calman, K. and Hine, D. (1995) Policy Framework for Commissioning Cancer Services: A Report by the Expert. Advisory Group on Cancer to the Chief Medical Officers of England and Wales. Available at www.dhcarenetworks.org.uk/_library/Resources/ICN/Policy_documents/Calman_Hine.pdf, accessed 22 October 2013.

Carerstrust. Available at www.carers.org/what-carer, accessed 21 May 2013.

Chan, D., Ong, B., Zhang, K., Li, R., Liu, J., Iedema, R. and Braithwaite, J. (2003) 'Hospitalisation, care plans and not for rescuscitation orders in older people in the last year of life.' *Age and Ageing 32*, 445–449.

Chaplin D. 'The Birmingham Bereavement Project: Executive Summary, June 2012.' Available at http://hoe.ioko.com/upload/PDFs/EXECUTIVE%20SUMMARY%20-%20The_Birmingham_Bereavement_Project%20Final.pdf.

Cicely Saunders Foundation (2011) 'About palliative care.' Available at www.cicelysaundersfoundation.org/about-palliative-care, accessed 21 May 2013.

Cicirelli, V. (2001) 'Personal meanings of death in older adults and young adults in relation to their fears of death.' *Death Studies 25*, 663–583.

Clark, D. (1993) 'Death in Staithes.,' In D. Dickenson and M. Johnson (eds) *Death, Dying and Bereavement.* London: Sage/Open University Press.

Clark, D. (2007) 'From margins to centre: A review of the history of palliative care in cancer.' *Lancet Oncology 8*, 430–438.

Connor, S.R., Egan, K.A., Kwilosz, D.M., Larson, D.G. and Reese, D.J. (2002) 'Interdisciplinary approaches to assisting with end-of-life care and decision making.' *American Behavioral Scientist 46*, 3, 340–356).

Coulshed, V. and Orme, J. (1998) *Social Work Practice: an introduction*, 3rd edition. Basingstoke: Macmillan.

Co-operative Funeralcare (2011) 'The way we say goodbye.' Available at www.co-operative. coop/Funeralcare/PDFs/Ways%20We%20Say%20Goodbye%20Brochure.pdf, accessed 21 May 2013.

Cruse Bereavement Care. 'Bereavement and older people.' Available at www.cruse.org.uk/sites/default/files/default_images/pdf/Documents-and-fact-sheets/OlderPeople.pdf, accessed 29 June 2013.

Curtis, J.R., Patrick, D.L. and Engelberg, R.A. (2001) 'Evaluating the quality of dying and death.' *Journal of Pain and Symptom Management 22*, 3, 717–26.

Curtis, J.R and Shannon, S.E (2006) 'Transcending the silos: toward an interdisciplinary approach to end-of-life care in the ICU.' *Intensive Care Medicine 32*, 1, 15–17.

Davie, G. (2007). *The Sociology of Religion.* London: Sage.

Dennis, J. (2013) 'Hospice: end-of-life conversations when the end is in sight.' Available at www.huffingtonpost.com/jeanne-dennis/end-of-life-planning_b_2633693.html?utm_hp_ref=tw, accessed 21 May 2013.

Department of Health (2006a) 'Our health our care our say.' Available at www.Department of Health.gov.uk/en/Publicationsandstatistics/Publications/PublicationsPolicyAndGuidance/Department of Health_4127602, accessed 21 May 2013.

Department of Health (2006b) 'Launch of dignity in care.' Available at www.Department of Health. gov.uk/en/Publicationsandstatistics/Lettersandcirculars/Dearcolleagueletters/Department of Health_063418, accessed 21 May 2013.

Department of Health (2008a) 'End of Life Care Strategy – promoting high quality care for all adults at the end of life.' Available at www.Department of Health.gov.uk/en/Publicationsandstatistics/Publications/PublicationsPolicyAndGuidance/Department of Health_086277, accessed 21 May 2013.

Department of Health (2008b) (February) 'Better Care Better Lives.' Available at www.Department of Health.gov.uk/en/Publicationsandstatistics/Publications/PublicationsPolicyAndGuidance/Department of Health_083106, accessed 21 May 2013.

Department of Health (2009) 'End of life care strategy: quality markers and measures for end of life care.' Available at www.Department of Health.gov.uk/en/Publicationsandstatistics/Publications/PublicationsPolicyAndGuidance/Department of Health_101681, accessed 21 May 2013.

Department of Health (2010) 'No decision about me, without me.' Available at http://www.dh.gov.uk/en/Publicationsandstatistics/Publications/PublicationsPolicyAndGuidance, accessed 23 October 2013.

Department of Health (2012a) 'Liberating the NHS: No decision about me, without me.' London: Crown Publications.

Detering, K., Hancock, A., Reade, M. and Silvester, W. (2010) 'The impact of advance care planning on end of life care in elderly patients: randomised controlled trial.' *British Medical Journal*, BMJ online 340 c1340.

Diane, T.E., Meier, Anthony. L., Back, R. and Morrison, S. (2001) 'The inner life of physicians and care of the seriously ill.' *Journal of American Medical Association 286*, 23, 3007–3014.

Dignity in Care, '10 point Dignity Challenge.' Available at www.dignityincare.org.uk/Dignity_in_Care_campaign/The_10_Point_Dignity_Challenge/, accessed 21 May 2013.

Dignity in Care Network. Available at www.dignityincare.org.uk, accessed 21 May 2013.

Draper, P., Holloway, M. and Adamson, S. (2013) 'A qualitative study of recently bereaved people's beliefs about death: Implications for bereavement care.' *Journal of Clinical Nursing.* doi: 10.1111/jocn.12326.

Dy, S.M., Shugarman, L.R., Lorenz, K.A., Mularski, R.A., Lynn, J. and for the RAND – Southern California Evidence-Based Practice Center (2008) 'A systematic review of satisfaction with care at the end of life'. *Journal of the American Geriatrics Society 56*, 1, 124–129.

Dying Matters (2013) 'Key facts.' Available at www.dyingmatters.org/overview/why-talk-about-it, accessed 21 May 2013.

Dying Matters 'Handling bereavement.' Available at www.dyingmatters.org/page/handling-bereavement, accessed 21 May 2013.

Economist Intelligence Unit (2010) *The Quality of Death: Ranking End of Life Care across the World.* Lien Foundation/Economist Intelligence Unit.

Elias, N. (1985) *The Loneliness of the Dying.* Oxford: Basil Blackwell.

Ellershaw, J., Murphy, D., Shea, T., Foster, A. and Overill, S. (1997) 'Developing an integrated pathway care pathway for the dying patient.' *European Journal of Palliative Care 4*, 203–208.

Ellershaw, J., Smith, C., Overill, S., Walker, S.E. and Aldridge, J. (2001) 'Care of the dying: setting standards for symptom control in the last 48 hours of life.' *Journal of Pain and Symptom Management 21*, 1, 12–17.

Ellershaw, J,. Dewar, S. and Murphy, D. (2010) 'Achieving a good death for all.' *British Medical Journal 341*, 656–658.

Ellershaw, J. and Wilkinson, S. (2011) *Care of the Dying: A pathway to excellence,* 2nd edition.' Oxford: Oxford University Press.

Engel, G. (1961) 'Is grief a disease?' *Psychosomatic Medicine 23*, 18–22.

Faber, S., Egnew, T. and Faber, A. (2004) 'What is a respectful death?' In J. Berzoff and P.R. Silverman (eds) *Living with Dying.* New York: Columbia University Press.

Fallowfield, L.J., Jenkins, V.A. and Beveridge, H.A. (2002) 'Truth may hurt but deceit hurts more: Communication in palliative care.' *Palliative Medicine 16*, 297–303.

Faull, C., de Castecker, S., Nicholson, A. and Black, F. (2012) *Handbook of Palliative Care.* London: John Wiley and Sons.

Ferrell, B.R. (2006) 'Understanding the moral distress of nurses witnessing medically futile care.' *Oncology Nursing Forum 33*, 5, 922–930.

Field, D. (1989) *Nursing the Dying.* London: Routledge.

Fleming, N.S. (2011) 'The financial and nonfinancial costs of implementing electronic health records in primary care practices.' *Health Affairs 30*, 3, 481–489.

Froggatt, K. (2001) 'Life and death within English nursing homes: sequestration of transition?' *Ageing and Society 21*, 319–332.

Gao, W., Ho, Y.K., Verne, J., Glickman, M. and Higginson, I. (2013) 'Changing patterns in place of cancer death in England: a population-based study.' *PLOS Medicine.* Available at www.plosmedicine.org/article/info:doi/10.1371/journal.pmed, accessed on 1 June 2013.

Gell, A. (1998) *Art and Agency: An Anthropological Theory.* Oxford: Clarendon.

General Medical Council (2011) 'Glossary of terms, end of life care.' Available at www.gmc-uk. org/guidance/ethical_guidance/end_of_life_glossary_of_terms.asp, accessed 21 May 2013.

General Medical Council (2013) 'Advance care planning.' Available at www.gmc-uk.org/guidance/ ethical_guidance/consent_guidance_advanced_care_planning.asp, accessed 21 May 2013.

George, R. (2011a) 'Truth telling, deceit and lying in cases of advanced dementia.' *End of Life Journal 1*, 1, 1–4.

George, R. (2011b) 'Exploring in more depth issues of truth telling, deceit and lying.' *End of Life Journal 1*, 2, 1–4.

Gerrard, R., Campbell, J., Minton, O., Moback, B. *et al.* (2010) 'Achieving the preferred place of care for hospitalized patients at the end of life.' *Palliative Medicine 25*, 4, 333–336.

Glaser, B. and Strauss, A. (1965) *Awareness of Dying.* Chicago: Aldine Publishing Co.

Glaser, B. and Strauss, A. (1967) *Time for Dying.* Chicago: Aldine Publishing Co.

Gomes, B. and Higginson, I. (2009) 'Where people die (1970–2030): past trends, future projections and implications for care.' *Palliative Medicine 22*, 1, 33–41.

Gomes, B., Calanzani, N. and Higginson, I.J. (2011) *Local Preferences and place of death in regions within England 2010.* London: Cicely Saunders International.

Gomes, B., Calanzani, N. and Higginson, I.J (2012a) 'Reversal of the British trends in place of death: Time series analysis 2004–2010.' *Palliative Medicine 26*, 2, 102–107.

Gomes, B., Higginson, I.J., Calanzani, N., Cohen, J., *et. al* (2012b) 'Preferences for place of death if faced with advanced cancer: A population survey in England, Flanders, Germany, Italy, the Netherlands, Portugal and Spain.' *Annals of Oncology* 23, 2006–2015.

Gorer, G. (1965), *Death, Grief and Mourning in Contemporary Britain.* London: Cresset Press.

Gott, M., Seymour, J., Bellamy, G., Clark, D. and Ahmedzai, S. (2004) 'Older people's views about home as a place of care at the end of life.' *Palliative Medicine*, 18, 460–467.

Gott, M., Small, N., Barnes, S., Payne, S. and Seamark, D. (2008) 'Older people's views of a good death in heart failure: Implications for palliative care provision.' *Social Science and Medicine 67*, 7, 1113–1121.

Grainger, R. (1998) *The Social Symbolism of Grief and Mourning.* London: Jessica Kingsley Publishers.

Grande, G., Addington-Hall, J. and Todd, C. (1998) 'Place of death and access to home care services: Are certain patient groups at a disadvantage?' *Social Science and Medicine 47*, 5, 565–579.

Grassi, L.T., Giraldi, E.G., Messina, K., and Magnani, E. *et al.* (2000) 'Physicians' attitudes to and problems with truth-telling to cancer patients.' *Supportive Care in Cancer 8*, 1, 40–45.

Harding R., Simon, S.T., Benalia, H., Downing, J. et al. (2011) 'PRISMA. The PRISMA Symposium 1: outcome tool use. Disharmony in European outcomes research for palliative and advanced disease care: too many tools in practice.' *Journal of Pain and Symptom Management 42*, 4, 493–500.

Higginson, I.J., Jarman, B., Astin, P. and Dolan, S. (1999). 'Do social factors affect where patients die: an analysis of 10 years of cancer deaths.' *Journal of Public Health Medicine 21*, 22–28.

Higginson, I.J. and Costantini, M. (2002) 'Communication in End-of-Life Cancer Care: A Comparison of Team Assessments in Three European Countries.' *Journal of Clinical Oncology 20*, 17, 3674–3682.

Higginson, I. and Gysels, M. (2000, 2003) *Improving supportive and palliative care for adults with cancer: Research Evidence Manual.* Available at http://www.nice.org.uk/nicemedia/pdf/ supportivepalliative_research_evidence_secondcons.pdf, accessed on 28 October 2013.

Hinton, J. (1972) *Dying*, 2nd edition. Harmondsworth: Penguin.

Hinton, J. (1980) 'Whom do dying patients tell?' *British Medical Journal 281*, 1328–30.

Hockey, J. (1990) *Experiences of Death: An Anthropological Account.* Edinburgh: Edinburgh University Press.

Hockey, J., Komaromy, C. and Woodthorpe, K. (2010) *The Matter of Death: Space, Place and Materiality.* Basingstoke: Palgrave Macmillan.

Hollis, F. (1972) *Casework : a psychosocial therapy,* 2nd edition. New York: Random House.

Holloway, M. (2007) *Negotiating Death in contemporary Health and Social Care.* Bristol: Policy Press.

Holloway, M. (2009) 'Dying old in the twenty-first century.' *International Social Work 52,* 6, 713–725.

Holloway, M. and Moss, B. (2010) *Spirituality and Social Work.* Basingstoke: Palgrave Macmillan.

Holloway, M., Adamson, S., McSherry, W. and Swinton, J. (2011) 'Spiritual care at the end of life: A systematic review of the literature.' London: Department of Health. Available at www.Department of Health.gov.uk/en/Publicationsandstatistics/Publications/ PublicationsPolicyAndGuidance/Department of Health_123812, accessed on 22 October 2013.

Holloway, M., Adamson, S., Argyrou, V., Draper, P. and Mariau, D. (2013) '"Funerals aren't nice but it couldn't have been nicer": The makings of a good funeral.' *Mortality 18,* 1, 30–53.

Holloway, M. and Taplin, S. (2013) 'Editorial: death and social work – 21st century challenges.' *British Journal of Social Work 43,* 2, 203–215.

Home Secretary and Secretary of State for Health (2007) 'Learning from tragedy, keeping patients safe.' Available at www.official-documents.gov.uk/document/cm70/7014/7014.pdf, accessed 21 May 2013.

Howarth, G. (1998) '"Just live for today." Living, caring, ageing and dying.' *Ageing and Society 18,* 673–689.

Hudson, P. (2004) 'Positive aspects and challenges associated within caring for a dying relative at home.' *International Journal of Palliative Nursing 10,* 2, 58–65.

Hughes, M. (2013) 'Decriminalising expected deaths in the home. A social work response.' *British Journal of Social Work 43,* 2, 282–297.

Hunwick, L., Juwle, S. and Mitchell, G. (2010) 'Symptom control at the end of life.' In P. Jevon, (ed.) *Care of the Dying and Deceased Patient.* Chichester: Wiley-Blackwell.

Institute of Healthcare Management (2010) *The National End of Life Care Programme's Communication Skills Pilot Project: an Independent Evaluation.* National End of Life Care Programme. Available at ihm.org.uk, accessed on 1 June 2013.

Institute of Healthcare Management (2011) *Advance Care Planning Implementation: Final Report.* National End of Life Care Programme. Available at ihm.org.uk, accessed on 1 June 2013.

Institute of Medicine (2001) *Crossing the Quality Chasm: A New Health System for the 21st Century.* Washington: National Academies of Sciences.

Institute of Medicine (2003) *Describing Death in America: What We Need to Know.* Washington: National Academies of Sciences.

Ipsos MORI (2011) 'End of life. Locality registers evaluation. Final report.' Available at www. endoflifecare.nhs.uk/search-resources/resources-search/publications/end-of-life-locality-registers-evaluation-final.aspx, accessed on 31 March 2013

Johns, C. (2006) *Engaging Reflection in Practice.* London: Blackwell Publishing.

Johnson S. (2007) 'Hope in terminal illness: An evolutionary concept analysis.' *International Journal of Palliative Nursing 13,* 9, 451–459.

Jordon, J. and Neimeyer, R. (2003) 'Does grief counselling work?' *Death Studies 27,* 9, 765–786.

Kadushin, A. and Kadushin, G. (2013) *The Social Work Interview: A Guide for Human Professionals,* 5th ed. New York: Columbia University Press.

Kane, R. (2003) 'The interface of long-term care and other components of health and social services systems in North America.' In J. Brodsky, J. Habib, and M. Hirschfield (eds) *Key Policy Issues in Long Term Care.* Geneva: World Health Organization Collaborating Centre for Research in Health in the Elderly, pp. 63–90.

Kanitsaki, O. (2002) 'Cultural perceptions and practices in dying, death and grieving. Conference report: Dying, Death and Grieving: A Cultural Perspective.' 22–23 March 2002. Australian Multicultural Foundation Aged Care Training Institute. Available at http://amf.net.au/library/uploads/files/Dying_Death_and_Grief_Conf.pdf, accessed on 30 April 2013.

Kellehear, A. (2005) *Compassionate Cities. Public health and end of life care.* London: Routledge.

Kellehear, A. (2007) *A Social History of Dying.* Cambridge: Cambridge University Press.

Kelly, B., McClement, S. and Chochinov, H. (2006) 'Measurement of psychological distress in palliative care.' *Palliative Medicine,* 20 (8), 779–789.

Kiehlmann, P. and Williamson, M. (2009) 'Anticipatory care planning – frequently asked questions.' Healthier Scotland/Scottish Government. Available at www.knowledge.scot. nhs.uk, accessed on 22 October 2013.

Kirsch, N. (2009) 'The Multidisciplinary Team: End-of-Life Ethical Decisions.' *Topics in Geriatric Rehabilitation 25*, 4, 292– 306.

Klass, D., Silverman, P.R. and Nickman, S. (1996) *Continuing Bonds: New Understanding of Grief.* London: Taylor & Francis.

Klinkenberg, M., Visser, G., Van Groenou, M., Van der Wal, G., Deeg, D. and Willems, D. (2005) 'The last 3 months of life: care, transitions and the place of death of older people.' *Health and Social Care in the Community 13*, 5, 420–430.

Knauft, E., Neilson, E., Engleberg, R., Donald, P. and Curtis, R. (2005) 'Barriers and facilitators to end-of-life care communication for patients with COPD.' *Ethics in Cardiopulmonary Medicine 127*, 6, 2188–2196.

Komaromy, C. (2000) 'The sight and sound of death: the management of dead bodies in residential and nursing homes.' *Mortality 5*, 3, 299–315.

Kramer, B.J. and Yonker, J.A. (2011) 'Perceived success in addressing end-of-life care needs of low-income elders and their families: what has family conflict got to do with it.' *Journal of Pain and Symptom Management 41*, 1, 35–48.

Kübler-Ross, E. (1969) *On Death and Dying.* London: Routledge.

Larson, D. and Tobin, D. (2000) 'End of life conversations: evolving theory and practice.' *Journal of the American Medical Association 284*, 12, 1573–1578.

Lawton, J. (2000) *The Dying Process: Patients' Experiences of Palliative Care.* London: Routledge.

Lloyd, M. [M. Holloway] and Taylor, C. (1995) 'From Hollis to the Orange Book: Developing a Holistic Model of Social Work Assessment in the 1990s.' *British Journal of Social Work 25*, 6, 691–710.

Lloyd, M. [M. Holloway] (1997) 'Dying and bereavement, spirituality and social work in a market economy of welfare.' *British Journal of Social Work 27*, 2, 175–190.

Long, C.O. (2011) 'Ten best practices to enhance culturally competent communication in palliative care.' *Journal of Paediatric Haematology/Oncology 33*, 2, 136–139.

Lord, B. and Pockett, R. (1998) 'Perceptions of social work intervention with bereaved clients: some implications for hospital social work practice.' *Social Work in Health Care 27*, 1, 51–66.

Machin, L. (2007) 'Resilience and Bereavement.' In B. Monroe and D. Oliviere (eds) *Resilience in Palliative Care – Achievement in Adversity.* Oxford: Oxford University Press, pp.157–165.

Macmillan Cancer Support (2012a) 'Over a million cancer carers miss out on vital support.' Available at www.macmillan.org.uk/Aboutus/News/Latest_News/ Overamillioncancercarersmissoutonvitalsupport.aspx, accessed 21 May 2013.

Macmillan Cancer Support (2012b) 'Hello and how are you? A guide for carers.' Available at www. macmillan.org.uk/Documents/HowWeCanHelp/HelloAnDepartment of HealthowAreYou.pdf, accessed 21 May 2013.

Macmillan Cancer Support (2013a) 'Not Alone Campaign.' Available at www.macmillan.org.uk/ Aboutus/OurNotAlonecampaign/Ournotalonecampaign.aspx, accessed 21 May 2013.

Macmillan Cancer Support (2013b) 'Facing the fight alone.' Available at www.macmillan.org.uk/ Documents/AboutUs/MAC13970_Isolated_cancer_patients_media_reportFINAL.pdf, accessed 21 May 2013.

Marie Curie Cancer Care (2003) 'Spiritual and religious care competencies for specialist palliative care.' Available at www.ahpcc.org.uk/pdf/spiritcomp.pdf, accessed 21 May 2013.

Marie Curie Delivering Choice Programme. Available at www.mariecurie.org.uk/deliveringchoice, accessed 21 May 2013.

Mason, C. (ed.) (2002) *Journeys into Palliative Care*. London: Jessica Kingsley Publishers.

McIlfatrick, S. (2007) 'Assessing palliative care needs: views of patients, informal carers and healthcare professionals.' *Journal of Advanced Nursing 57*, 1, 77–86.

Mental Health Law Online. Available at www.mentalhealthlaw.co.uk/Mental_Capacity_Act_2005, accessed 21 May 2013.

Ministry of Justice (2012) 'A guide to coroners and inquests and charter for coroner services.' Available at www.justice.gov.uk/coroners-burial-cremation/coroners, accessed 21 May 2013.

Monroe, B. (2004) 'Social work in palliative medicine.' In D. Doyle, G. Hanks and N.I. Cherny (eds) *Oxford Textbook of Palliative Medicine* (3rd edition). Oxford: Oxford University Press.

Morris, J. (2012) 'Integrated care for frail older people 2012: a clinical overview.' *Journal of Integrated Care 20*, 4, 257–264.

Munday, D., Dale, J. and Murray, S. (2007) 'Choice and place of death: individual preferences, uncertainty, and the availability of care.' *Journal of the Royal Society of Medicine 100*, 5. 211–215.

National Association of Social Workers (NASW). Available at www.naswdc.org, accessed 21 May 2013.

National Audit Office (2008) *Report on End of Life*. London: Crown.

National Cancer Action Team (2010) 'Characteristics of effective MDT working.' Available at http://ncat.nhs.uk/sites/default/files/NCATMDTCharacteristics.pdf, accessed 21 May 2013.

National Council for Palliative Care/National End Of Life Care Programme (2013) 'Advance decisions to refuse treatment – a guide for health and social care professionals.' Available at www.endoflifecare.nhs.uk/search-resources/resources-search/publications/imported-publications/advance-decisions-to-refuse-treatment.aspx, accessed 21 May 2013.

National End of Life Care Intelligence Network (2010) *Deaths from Alzheimer's Disease, Dementia and Senility in England*. London: NEoLCIN.

National End of Life Care Intelligence Network (2012) *What Do We Know Now that We Didn't Know a Year Ago?* London: NEoLCIN.

National End of Life Care Programme (2008) *Advance Care Planning: A Guide for Health and Social Care Staff, revised version*. London: Department of Health. Available online at www.endoflifecare. nhs.uk, accessed 31 March 2013.

National End of Life Care Programme (2009a) *Planning for Your Future Care: a Guide*. Leicester: National End of Life Care Programme.

National End of Life Care Programme (2009b) *Common Core Competences and Principles for End of Life Care*. Leicester: National End of Life Care Programme.

National End of Life Care Programme (2010a) 'Holistic common assessment of supportive and palliative care needs for adults requiring palliative and end of life care.' NEoLCP/National Cancer Action Team. Available at www.nhsiq.nhs.uk/resource-search/publications/eolc-hca-guide.aspx, accessed on 25 September 2013.

National End of Life Care Programme (2010b) 'Talking needs action, training needs analysis.' Available at www.endoflifecare.nhs.uk/search-resources/resources-search/publications/importedpublications/talking-needs-action-training-needs-analysis.aspx, accessed 21 May 2013.

National End of Life Care Programme (2010c) 'Supporting people to live and die well – a framework for social care at the end of life.' Available at www.nhsiq.nhs.uk/resource-search/publications/eolc-supporting-people-to-live-and-die-well.aspx, accessed 25 September 2013.

National End of Life Care Programme (2010d) *The Route to Success in End of Life Care – Achieving Quality in Acute Hospitals*. London: Crown Copyright.

National End of Life Care Programme (2011a) 'The route to success in end of life care – achieving quality for people with learning disabilities.' Available at www.nhsiq.nhs.uk/resource-search/publications/eolc-rts-learning-disabilities.aspx, accessed 25 September 2013.

National End of Life Care Programme (2011b) *Critical Success Factors that Enable Individuals to Die in Their Preferred Place of Death*. Leicester: National End of Life Care Programme.

National End of Life Care Programme (2011c) *Guidance for Staff Responsible for Care after Death.* Leicester: National End of Life Care Programme.

National End of Life Care Programme (2011d) *Draft Spiritual Support and Bereavement Care Quality Markers and Measures for End of Life Care.* Leicester: National End of Life Care Programme.

National End of Life Care Programme (2011e) *Route to Success: the Key Contribution of Nursing to End of Life Care.* London: Crown Publications.

National End of Life Care Programme (2012a) 'The route to success in end of life care – achieving quality for lesbian, gay, bisexual and transgender people.' Available at www.nhsiq.nhs.uk/resource-search/publications/eolc-rts-lgbt.aspx, accessed 25 September 2013.

National End of Life Care Programme (2012b) 'The route to success in end of life care – achieving quality for social work.' Available at http://www.nhsiq.nhs.uk/resource-search/publications/eolc-rts-social-work.aspx, accessed 25 September 2013.

National End of Life Care Programme (2012c) 'Advance care planning: it all ADSE up.' Available at www.nhsiq.nhs.uk/resource-search/publications/eolc-acp-guide.aspx, accessed 25 September 2013.

National End of Life Care Programme (2012d) 'Optimising the role and value of the interdisciplinary team: Providing person-centred end of life care.' National End of Life Care Programme. Available at www.endoflifecare.nhs.uk, accessed 31 March 2013.

National End of Life Care Programme (2012e) 'Electronic Palliative Care Coordination Systems (EPaCCS) mid 2012 survey report.' Available at www.endoflifecare.nhs.uk/search-resources/resources-search/publications/epaccs-mid-2012-survey-report.aspx, accessed on 31st March 2013.

National End of Life Care Programme (2012f) 'Making the case for change – Electronic Palliative Care Co-ordination Systems.' Available at www.nhsiq.nhs.uk/resource-search/publications/eolc-epaccs-case-for-change.aspx, accessed 25 September 2013.

National End of Life Care Programme (2013) 'The Route to Success series.' Available at www.nhsiq.nhs.uk/resource-search/publications.aspx?pb=3841&rpp=5&sortby=Latest, accessed 25 September 2013.

National End of Life Care Programme (2012) 'Transforming end of life care in acute hospitals: Overview and progress update December 2012.' Available at www.endoflifecare.nhs.uk/search-resources/resources-search/publications/imported-publications/transforming-end-of-life-care-in-acutehospitals.aspx, accessed 21 May 2013.

National End of Life Care Programme/Housing Learning and Improvement Network (2012) 'End of life care in extra care housing – learning resource pack for housing, care and support staff' Available at www.endoflifecare.nhs.uk/search-resources/resources-search/publications/learning-resource-pack-eolc-in-extra-care-housing.aspx, accessed 21 May 2013.

National End of Life Care Programme/NHS Improvement (2010) 'End of life care in heart failure. A framework for implementation.' Available at www.endoflifecare.nhs.uk/search-resources/resourcessearch/publications/imported-publications/end-of-life-care-in-heart-failure.aspx.

National Council for Palliative Care (2011) Capacity, Care Planning And Advance Care Planning In Life Limiting Illness. Available at http://www.ncpc.org.uk/freedownloads, accessed 23 October 2013.

National Institute for Clinical Excellence (NICE) (2004) *Guidance on Cancer Services: Improving Supportive and Palliative Care for Adults with Cancer: The Manual.* London: National Institute for Clinical Excellence.

National Institute for Health and Care Excellence (NICE) (2011) 'Quality standard for end of life care.' Available at http://publications.nice.org.uk/quality-standard-for-end-of-life-care-for-adults-qs13, accessed 21 May 2013.

National Institutes of Health. *National Institutes of Health State-of-the-Science Conference: Statement on Improving End-of-Life Care.* 6-8 December 2004. 4 November 2006. Available at http://consensus.nih.gov/2004/2004EndOfLifeCareSOS024html.htm, accessed on 22 October 2013.

Neale, D. (2010) *Establishing the Extra in Extra Care. Perspectives from Three Extra Care Housing Providers.* London: International Longevity Centre UK.

Nelson, J. (2006) 'Identifying and overcoming the barriers to high-quality palliative care in the intensive care unit.' *Critical Care Medicine 34*, 11, 324–331.

Neuberger, J. (2004) *Dying Well: a Guide to Enabling a Good Death.* 2nd ed. Oxford: Radcliffe Publishing.

Ngo-Metzger, Q., August, K.J., Srinivasan, M., Liao, S., and Meyskens, F.L.Jr. (2008) 'End-of life care: guidelines for patient-centered communication.' *American Family Physician 77*, 2, 167–174.

NHS Information Standards Board. 'End of life care co-ordination: core content.' Available at www.isb.nhs.uk/library/standard/236, accessed 21 May 2013.

NHS Interoperability Toolkit. Available at www.connectingforhealth.nhs.uk/systemsandservices/interop, accessed 21 May 2013.

Nolan, S. and Holloway, M. (in press) *An A–Z of Spirituality for the Caring Professions.* Basingstoke: Palgrave Macmillan.

Nuland, S. (1995) *How We Die.* New York: Vintage Books, Random House.

O'Connor, S.J. (2008) 'End of life care definitions and triggers to assessment: a summary and discussion of the literature.' Available at www.endoflifecare.nhs.uk/assets/downloads/EOLC_Literature_Review_Oct2008.pdf, accessed 21 May 2013.

Oliver, D. (ed.) (2012) *End of Life Care in Neurological Disease.* London: Springer.

Ong, C.-K. and Forbes, D. (2005) 'Embracing Cicely Saunders' concept of total pain.' *British Medical Journal 331*, 7516, 576–577.

Oxford Dictionary (2013) Available at http://oxforddictionaries.com/definition/english/holistic, accessed 21 May 2013.

Paddy, M. (2011) 'Influence of location on a good death.' *Nursing Standard 26*, 1, 33–36.

Parker, J. (ed) (2005) *Aspects of Social Work and Palliative Care.* London: Quay Books.

Parker, J. and Bradley, G. (2010) *Social work practice: assessment, planning, intervention and review*, 3rd edition. Exeter: Learning Matters.

Parkes, C.M. (1975) *Bereavement: Studies of Grief in Adult Life.* London: Penguin.

Parkes, C.M. (1998) 'Coping with loss: bereavement in adult life.' *British Medical Journal 316*, 7134, 856–859.

Pattison, N. (2011) 'Organ Donation.' In M. Baldwin and J. Woodhouse (eds) *Key Concepts in Palliative Care*, pp.121–126. London: Sage.

Paul, S. (2013) 'Public health approaches to palliative care: the role of the hospice social worker working with children experiencing bereavement.' *British Journal of Social Work 43*, 2, 249–263.

Payne, M. (2007) 'Know your colleagues – role of social work in end of life care.' *End of Life Care 1*, 1, 69–73.

Payne, M. (2012) 'Palliative care social work competencies: they need to show social work is social.' Available at http://blogs.stchristophers.org.uk/one/, accessed 21 May 2013.

Pelletier, L.R. and Beaudin, C. (2008) *Q Solutions: Essential Resources for the Healthcare Quality Professional, Second Edition.* Glenview, IL: National Association for Healthcare Quality.

Pickering, M., Littlewood, J. and Walter, T. (1997) 'Beauty and the beast: sex and death in the tabloid press.' In D. Field, J. Hockey and N. Small (eds) *Death, Gender and Ethnicity.* London: Routledge.

Public Health England. 'End of Life Care Quality Assessment Tool (ELQuA).' Available at www.elcqua.nhs.uk/, accessed 21 May 2013.

Rabow, M.W., Hauser, J.M., and Adams, J. (2004) 'Supporting family caregivers at the end of life: "They don't know what they don't know".' *JAMA: The Journal of the American Medical Association, 291*, 4, 483–491.

Raftery, J.P., Addington-Hall, J.M., MacDonald, L.D., Anderson, H.R. et al. (1996) 'A randomized controlled trial of the cost-effectiveness of a district co-ordinating service for terminally ill cancer patients.' *Palliative Medicine: Sage Journals 10*, 2, 151–161.

Ratner, E., Norlander, L. and McSteen, K. (2001) 'Death at home following a targeted advance care planning process at home: the kitchen table discussion.' *American Geriatric Society*, 49, 778–81.

Reb, A. (2003) 'Palliative and end-of-life care: policy analysis.' *Oncology Nursing Forum 30*, 1, 35–50.

Reith, M. and Payne, M. (2009) *Social Work in End of Life and Palliative Care.* Bristol: Policy Press.

Relf, M. (2008) 'Risk Assessment and Bereavement Services.' In S.A. Payne, J. Seymour, J. Skilbeck and C. Ingleton (eds) *Palliative Care Nursing: Principles and Evidence for Practice.* Buckingham: Open University Press.

Relf, M., Machin, L. and Archer, N. (2010) *Guidance for Bereavement Needs Assessment in Palliative Care*, 2nd edition. London: Help the Hospices. Available at www.helpthehospices.org.uk, accessed 25 September 2013.

Richardson, A., Sitzia, J., Brown, V., Medina, J., Richardson, A. (2005) *Patients' Needs Assessment Tools in Cancer Care: Principles and Practice.* London: King's College London.

Rickerson, E. (2005) 'Prevalence of grief-related symptoms and need for bereavement support among long term care staff.' *Journal of Pain and Symptom Management 30*, 3, 227–233.

Royal College of Nursing (RCN) (2011) 'The End of Life Patient Charter.' Available at www.rcn. org.uk/data/assets/pdf_file/0005/386888/EOLC_Charter_FINAL_for_launch_2011_06_01. pdf, accessed 21 May 2013.

Royal College of Physicians (RCP). Available at www.rcplondon.ac.uk, accessed 21 May 2013.

Saunders, C. (ed.) (1990) *Hospice and Palliative Care: An Interdisciplinary Approach.* London: Edward Arnold.

SCIE (2013) Report 37: 'Personalisation, productivity and efficiency.' Available at www.scie.org.uk/publications/reports/report37/index.asp, accessed 21 May 2013.

Seale, C. (1995) 'Dying alone.' *Sociology of Health and Illness 17*, 377–391.

Seale, C. and Cartwright, A. (1994) *The Year Before Death.* Aldershot: Avebury.

Selman, L., Harding, R., Speck, P., Robinson, V., Aguma, A., Rys, A., Kyei-Baffour, N. and Higginson, I. (2010) *Spiritual Care Recommendations for People from Black and Minority Ethnic (BME) Groups Receiving Palliative Care in the UK.* London: Cicely Saunders Foundation/Sir Halley Stewart Trust.

Selwyn, P. (2008) 'Commentary: palliative care and social justice.' *Journal of Pain and Symptom Management 36*, 5, 513–515.

Shannon, S.E., Long-Sutehall, T. and Coombs, M. (2011) 'Conversations in end-of-life care: communication tools for critical care practitioners.' *Nursing in Critical Care 16*, 3, 124–130.

Sheehy, L. (2013) 'Understanding factors that influence the grieving process.' *End of Life Care Journal 3*, 1.

Sheldon, F. (1997) *Psychosocial Palliative Care.* Cheltenham: Stanley Thornes.

Shipman, C., Gysels, M., White, P., Worth, A. *et al.* (2008) 'Improving generalist end of life care: national consultation with practitioners, commissioners, academics, and service user groups.' *British Medical Journal 1*, doi: 10.1136/bmj.a1720.

Skilbeck, J.K. and Payne, S. (2005) 'End of life care: a discursive analysis of a specialist in palliative care nursing.' *Journal of Advanced Nursing 51*, 4, 325–334.

Smith, T. (2011) 'Why social workers need to talk about death' [blog]. Available at www.communitycare.co.uk/blogs/adult-care-blog/2011/05/why-social-workers-need-to-talk-about-death.html, accessed 21 May 2013.

Smith, T. and Sherwen, E. (2012) 'End of Life Care.' In D. Oliver (ed.) (2012) *End of Life Care in Neurological Disease.* London: Springer.

Spencer, N. and Weldin, H. (2012) *Post-religious Britain? The faith of the faithless.* Theos: London. Available at http://www.theosthinktank.co.uk/files/files/Post%20Religious%20Britain%20pdf. pdf, accessed on 30 September 2013.

South West Public Health Observatory. Available at www.swpho.nhs.uk/, accessed 21 May 2013.

Stroebe, M. and Schut, H. (1999) 'The dual process model of coping with bereavement: rationale and description.' *Death Studies 23,* 197–224.

Stroebe, M., Hansson, R., Stroebe, W. and Schut, H. (2001) *Handbook of Bereavement Research: Consequences, Coping and Care.* Washington DC: American Psychological Association.

Stroebe, M.S., Folkman, S., Hansson, R.O. and Schut, H. (2006) 'The prediction of bereavement outcome: development of an integrative risk factor framework.' *Social Science and Medicine 63,* 2440–2451.

Sturmberg, J.P., O'Halloran, D.M. and Martin, C.M. (2012) 'Understanding health system reform – a complex adaptive systems perspective.' *Journal of Evaluation in Clinical Practice 18,* 1, 202–208.

Sudnow, D. (1967) *Passing On: The Social Organization of Dying.* New York: Prentice Hall.

Surbone, A. (2011) 'Effect of cultural and socioeconomic factors on acceptance and delivery of palliative and end of life care.' *American Society of Clinical Oncology,* Education Book, 111–115.

Sykes, N. (2012) 'Care at the End of Life.' In D. Oliver (ed.) *End of Life in Neurological Disease.* London: Springer.

The Lancet Editorial (2011) 'Truth telling in clinical practice.' *The Lancet 378,* 9798, 1197.

The Quotations Page. Available at www.quotationspage.com/quote/31461.html, accessed 16 June 2013.

Thomas, K. (2003) *Caring for the Dying at Home: Companions on the Journey.* Milton Keynes: Radcliffe Publishing.

Thomas, K. and Lobo, B. (eds) (2011) *Advance Care Planning in End of Life Care.* Oxford: Oxford University Press.

Twycross, R. (1997) *Introducing Palliative Care,* 2nd ed. Abingdon: Radcliffe Medical Press.

Valentine, C. (2006) 'Academic constructions of bereavement.' *Mortality 11,* 1, 57–77.

Van Gennep, A. (1909, republished 1960) *The Rites of Passage.* Chicago: University of Chicago Press.

Voas, D., and Crockett, A. (2005). 'Religion in Britain: neither believing nor belonging.' *Sociology 39,* 1, 11–28.

Walker, N. (2012) 'Dying well: towards a community response.' Available at www.endoflifecare.nhs. uk, accessed on 31 March 2013.

Waller, S. (2008) *Improving Environments for Care at the End of Life: Lessons from Eight UK Pilot Programmes.* London: The King's Fund.

Walter, T. (1994) *The Revival of Death.* London: Routledge.

Walter, T. (1996) 'A new model of grief: bereavement and biography.' *Mortality 1,* 1, 7–25.

Walter, T. (1999) *On Bereavement: The Culture of Grief.* Buckingham: Open University Press.

Watson, M. (2010) 'Spiritual Aspects of Advance Care Planning.' In K. Thomas and B. Lobo (eds) *Advance Care Planning in End of Life Care.* Oxford: Oxford University Press.

Watts, T. (2012) 'End of life care pathway tools to promote a good death: a critical commentary.' *European Journal of Cancer Care 21,* 1, 20–30

Way, D., Jones, L. and Busing, N. (2000) 'Implementation Strategies: Collaboration in Primary Care - Family Doctors and Nurse Practitioners Delivering Shared Care.' Discussion paper written for the Ontario College of Family Physicians. Available at http://www.eicp.ca/en/toolkit/hhr/ ocfp-paper-handout.pdf, accessed 28 October 2013.

Weissman, D.E. and Meiler, D.E. (2011) 'Identifying patients in need of a palliative care assessment in the hospital setting – a consensus report from the center to advance palliative care.' *Journal of Palliative Medicine 14,* 1, 1–7.

Williams, R. (1990) *A Protestant Legacy: Attitudes to Death and Illness among Older Aberdonians.* Oxford: Clarendon Press.

Wilson, J. and Kirshbaum, M. (2011) 'Effects of patient death on nursing staff: A literature review.' *British Journal of Nursing 20*, 9, 559–563.

Wimpenny, P. (2006) *A Literature Review on Bereavement and Bereavement Care.* Aberdeen: The Robert Gordon University.

Woodhead, L. (2013) 'Changing rituals and meanings around death.' Welcome collection conference: 'What makes a good death?' 1–2 February 2013. Available at www.wellcomecollection.org, accessed on 1 June 2013.

Worden, J.W. (1991) *Grief Counselling and Grief Theory. A Handbook for the Mental Health Practitioner (2nd edition).* London: Routledge.

World Health Organization (1998) 'WHO Definition of Palliative Care.' Available at http://www.who.int/cancer/palliative/definition/en/, accessed 30 October 2013.

Wright, A.A., Zhang, B., Ray, A., Mack, J.W., Trice, E., Balboni, T., *et al.* (2008) 'Associations between end-of-life discussions, patient mental health, medical care near death, and caregiver bereavement adjustment.' *Journal of the American Medical Association 300*, 1665–1673.

von Gunten, C.F., Ferris, F.D. and Emanuel, L.L. (2000) 'Ensuring Competency in End-of-Life Care Communication and Relational Skills.' *JAMA 284*, 23, 3051–3057.

Young, M. and Cullen, L. (1996) *A Good Death: Conversations with East Londoners.* London: Routledge.

Subject Index

Author Index